Fresh Air and Streptomycin

Rosemary E Brown

ATHENA PRESS
LONDON

CW01390651

FRESH AIR AND STREPTOMYCIN
Copyright © Rosemary E Brown 2009

All Rights Reserved

ISBN 978 1 84748 626 4

First published 2009 by
ATHENA PRESS
Queen's House, 2 Holly Road
Twickenham TW1 4EG
United Kingdom

Every effort has been made to trace the copyright holders
of works quoted within this book and obtain permission.
The publisher apologises for any omission and is happy
to make necessary changes in subsequent print runs.

Printed for Athena Press

To: John

Fresh Air and Streptomycin

Best wishes

Rosemary Brown

February 2010

I dedicate this book to my dear father, George, and mother, Clara, whose love for me was unconditional, even through those dark, endless days with me, their only child, aged 5½, shut away from them in institutions and hospitals for twenty-two months.

Their suffering must have been far worse than mine, not knowing whether I would live or die. My dear, quiet, rustic and gentle dad, with his love of nature and animals, was my absolute 'soulmate' before my hospitalisation, and continued to be so after my return home. My mother was the strong leader of our little family, but being separated for so long in those formative years created an unavoidable gap between us, but I continued to love her very dearly all the same. Dad's death in 1991 and Mum's in 2008 took them to their graves knowing they had taken the right decision, and had trusted and put faith in the medical profession, in October 1947, to permit their only child, 'Rowy', to be treated with this unknown, untried and new antibiotic drug called streptomycin.

Note from the Author

I was born Rosemary Elizabeth Webb on 17 September 1941. I am now a pensioner and have decided that I must put down on paper my recollections of my near-terminal illness in 1947. I want to record my experiences of that most dreadful time, for my own sake and that of my parents and family.

The illness was miliary TB. I survived that illness thanks mostly to the American government, the soon-to-be-created NHS (which benefited me after my discharge), Bristol Hospital for Sick Children, Jan Smuts Home at Burnham-on-Sea, Dr Beryl Corner, the staff at Bristol and Burnham, and the new wonder drug streptomycin. Thanks also are expressed to the doctors and staff at both the County Hospital and Nieuport Sanatorium. A special thank you goes out to Dr Godfrey Malkin, our local GP, without whose 'pushing' for a bed for me to trial the drug I would not have survived.

It is still a mystery how I contracted this dreadful disease, but I lived to tell the tale and I have put my experiences into my own words over the next few chapters. My mother, Clara, before her death, helped me with timings and content.

Chapter 1

Parents and Grandparents

My father, George Arthur Webb, was born in 1911, the fifth and youngest child of Bryan Meredith and Elizabeth Webb. My father had a very traumatic life in his younger years. His father, Bryan, was killed in a steamroller accident on Bodcott Hill, near Bredwardine. He died on 16 April, when my father, George, was just ten months old.

Nearing the end of the millennium, on 31 December 1999, I located and visited the grave of Bryan in Kinnersley Churchyard. This little village is near Kington in Herefordshire. The writing on the gravestone reads:

In loving memory
BRYAN MEREDITH WEBB
April 16th 1912
Aged 36 years

I know not what awaits me
The path I cannot see
I left its toils and sorrows
With one who died with me.

This was the first time I had visited my grandfather's grave as, up until now, I did not know where my grandparents were buried. I still have no idea of the resting place of my grandmother, Elizabeth. Bryan died in the same week that the great ocean liner *Titanic* went to the bottom of the Atlantic Ocean with a great loss of life. The loss to my family of my grandfather was equally as important as the loss of lives on that great liner.

I am, even to this day, intrigued as to what he looked like. Was he like my dear dad, loving and giving? My father, George, was a friendly, loving, generous man. The Webb male line were not 'giants of men' but strong and loving. Dad was short in stature, as were his two brothers and two sisters.

I have been reliably informed that the steamroller in the picture (opposite) is an Aveling and Porter, with the motto of Kent on the front, i.e. *The Invicta*. The number of the engine is believed to be 4662.

I had always heard that Granddad Webb had been run over by a steamroller. In my childhood, I relayed the story to my school chums, revelling in the fact that he had met such a grisly end. Not many of my chums could boast of such family history, but, in truth, I did not know much about the event. My father had told me that his dad had had an accident and had died when he was ten months old and that was that... until the *Hereford Times* printed an extra booklet in December 1999 giving details of events over the previous one hundred years. There it was, with a picture: the details of how my grandfather had died. There was a report and a picture of the crippled steamroller stating that the fireman, Bryan Webb, had been seriously hurt in the accident.

I recently placed an appeal in the *Hereford Times* desperately seeking information about this most dreadful accident and asking if anyone had a photograph of Bryan. This, I thought, was like grasping at straws in the wind. A minimal response, if any, was expected.

My grandfather appeared to have been the hero of the day, staying on the crippled steamroller while it ran down Bodcott Hill. My father told me some years ago that apparently Bryan's mother, Elizabeth, was in the living van behind the steamroller and that Bryan was trying to save her life.

A few people responded to my appeal, one being a Mrs Column, who had the same photograph in her possession. She knew not how it had come to be with her, but it was a photograph made into a postcard. It seemed to have been the fashion in the early part of the twentieth century to turn everything into a postcard!

The writer on the back of the postcard had written:

> Fools boldly rush in
> Where angels fear to tread.

Two other people responded, one with photographs of a team of workmen at Weobley, but no definite photographs of Grandfather Webb. One gentleman, who lives in Hereford, is a steam enthusiast.

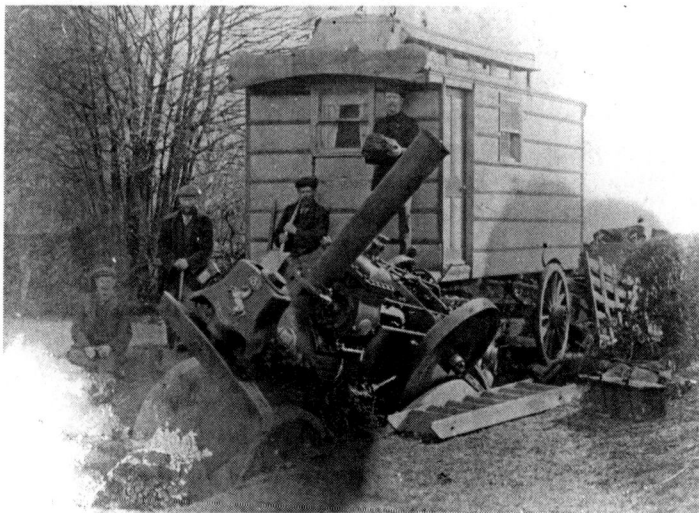

The steamroller accident

Going back to the time of grandfather's accident, the *Hereford Times* reports in its edition dated 19 April 1912:

On Wednesday afternoon of last week, a steamroller of Mr Chambers of Clifford, which was on hire to the Weobley District Council, had been rolling in the vicinity of Moccas and was proceeding along the road towards Bredwardine on its way to Kinnersley, when, in descending a steep hill, something is supposed to have happened to the steering gear. The roller got out of control, dashed through a gateway, tearing up the posts, and falling into a brook about six feet deep. The driver, William Lewis[*], seems to have escaped without much injury, but Bryan Webb who was the fireman got pinned between the living van and the engine and narrowly escaped being killed.

The *Hereford Times*, in a later edition, reports on the coroner's inquest into the untimely death of Grandfather Webb.

On Tuesday evening Bryan Webb, roadman of Kinnersley, died in the Herefordshire General Hospital as a result of injuries he received on April 3rd at Bredwardine. It will be remembered that, as stated in the *Hereford Times*, he was steering a traction engine down the Bodcott Pitch when the steering gear broke and the engine tore down the hill uncontrolled. In consequence of this, the engine turned over into the ditch, when the unfortunate man was pinned between the wagon and the hind wheel of the engine. He was subsequently brought to Hereford, but in spite of medical aid, his injuries terminated fatally.

The inquest was held at the Herefordshire General Hospital on Thursday afternoon before the City Coroner, Mr J Lambe, Mr J J Jones was foreman of the jury.

William Lewis, traction engine driver, Kinnersley, identified the body as that of his stepson Bryan Webb. Deceased was 36 years of age. He had worked on a road roller as a steerer for three years for the Weobley District

---

[*] William Lewis was Bryan Webb's stepfather.

Council. During the last ten years he had been a roadman. A fortnight on Wednesday, witness and Deceased were returning from Blakemere to Kinnersley. When they got to within half a mile of Bredwardine, they came to the Bodcott Pitch, where the fork of the roller broke. Deceased was steering at the time. As a result of this they lost control of the engine and owing to the weight behind them they could not stop it. After running with the steam shut off and the brakes applied, the engine ran into the ditch on the right-hand side of the road. Witness had his leg caught fast between front wheel of the wagon and the tender of the engine where he hung head downwards. When he got clear he found his stepson underneath the wagon with his left leg crushed between the fork of the drawbar and the hind wheel of the engine. Witness released his leg, when some people helped to carry him out of the wreckage. He was then removed home by Mr Wilson.

In reply to a juror, witness said he stuck to his post to the last. He did not jump off because he held the brakes, otherwise more injury might have been done.

Juror: You acted very properly.

The Coroner: What weight had you behind you?

Witness: About three and a half tons.

Mr Barrell: Was it an old engine?

Witness: I don't know, but it was passed by the Inspector twelve months ago.

Joseph Wilson, landlord of the Lion Hotel in Bredwardine, said he and his wife heard of the accident, and in response to a message they drove to Bodcott Hill where the injured man was found. Witness's wife, who had been a nurse, took with her bandages, pillows and other things to render first aid. Deceased was lying in the field on the other side of the hedge. His thigh was fractured and he was bleeding very much. Witness's wife bound up the leg and stopped the bleeding, after which witness drove the man home and despatched a man on horseback for Dr Steed. He should like to add, in consequence of rumours, that both men were perfectly sober. Mr de F Pennefather drove the injured man to Hereford in his car the next day.

A Juror: You acted the Good Samaritan, Mr Wilson.

Edward Symonds Chambers, Machinist, Clifford, owner of the engine said the fork of the engine was put in new three years ago. He bought it from London County Council four years ago, and it was in good order. It was passed by the Inspector for the purpose of insurance twelve months since.

Vincent Phillip Norman, house surgeon at the Herefordshire General Hospital, said Deceased was suffering from a compound fracture of the left thigh bone. The leg was put in splints and for four or five days the patient went on well, after which blood poisoning set in, followed by haemorrhage. The only chance of saving his life was an operation, and his leg was removed on April 16th. He never rallied after the operation and died on the evening of the 16th April. The cause of death was heart failure due to shock and blood poisoning.

A verdict of accidental death was returned.

The foreman of the jury said that he would like to express to Mr Wilson their sense of kindness he had extended to the injured man.

Mr Wilson thanked the jury. He said he knew the Deceased very well. He was a tidy, hardworking man and he was very sorry for his family. Deceased leaves behind him a widow and four little children, one of whom was stone blind.*

---

* This should read five children: William, Kathleen, Florence, Walter and George Arthur (my father).

My paternal grandmother, Elizabeth, was now a widow with five children to support, the youngest of them being my father, George, aged just ten months. He had four elder brothers and sisters. William (Bill) who was the 'stone' blind child referred to in the inquest, was the eldest boy.

Bill is said to have been playing with his cousin at home at Kinnersley Post Office, throwing hot ashes or lime about, when an accident occurred in which his eyes were burnt. This story varies throughout the family, but I would assume that it was lime, as hot ashes would not be so easy to handle. My father told me that his mother refused medical aid and Billy was placed in a home for the blind.

Elizabeth would have obviously been devastated by her young husband's death, and how she coped we do not know, but she remarried a man called Bill Candy and had a further child with him, a girl called Nina, my father's stepsister.

Further tragedy was to strike this family. During the 1918 great influenza epidemic, my grandmother Elizabeth died, having gone next door to nurse her neighbour. She unfortunately contracted the virus and died soon afterwards, leaving the unfortunate children as orphans, my father being the youngest at six years old.

My father told me he remembered the day of his mother's death, of relatives coming to 'sort things out'. He remembers his stepsister, Nina, being carried out of the house, crying in someone's arms. He did not know where she was going and did not ask as he was only six himself.

In those days, it was down to the family to 'sort things out', except for the eldest girl, Florrie, who was in service and the eldest boy, Billy (William) who was in a home for the blind. The rest were handed around like chattels to various family members. My father was taken by his Uncle George by bicycle to Cwms Wood, Bromyard, to live with Uncle George and his wife. George's wife was to die soon afterwards, leaving my father and Uncle George to live life as best they could on their own, with no woman to look after them. This, however, was infinitely better than the workhouse, which is where most orphans ended up. He worked very hard for his uncle.

My father lived at Cwms Wood until his teens, living a very unhappy and austere life, with little or no food. He recalled to me that during his shopping trips to Bromyard with the horse and cart he would eat some of the shopping on the way home, including raw sausages!

When he was about sixteen years old he left his 'foster' home at Cwms Wood and went to work at Munderfield, near Bromyard. He was there for about two years and then moved to another live-in job at Chapel Farm, How Caple, which was to be his home until his marriage.

Moving on to the maternal side of my family, Samuel Jones and his wife Ellen (née Gardiner) had a less fraught life, in that they enjoyed seeing their children grow into adulthood.

My mother, Clara Louisa Webb (née Jones), was born in 1914, the fourth child of Samuel and Ellen Jones.

Samuel and Ellen had eight children who lived, and one who died in childhood: Gladys, Cyril, Lewis, Clara (my mother), Florence, Marjorie, Charles, Francis (who died in childhood) and Frances.

My mother was given the names Clara Louisa and was not expected to live. She hated these names right up until her death and much preferred to be called Clare.

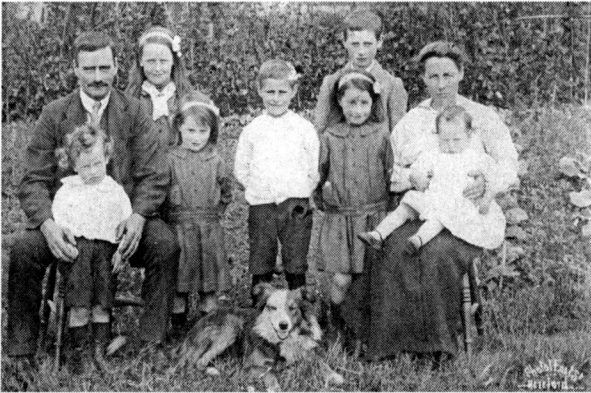

From left to right: Granddad Samuel Jones (seated), Charles, Gladys, Clara, Lewis, Cyril (back), Marjorie, Grandmother Ellen Jones, Frances (on lap) and Scottie the dog (Florence is missing from the photograph.)

My grandfather, Samuel Jones, was a farm worker, but was an equally good mechanic and was self-taught. He was always tinkering with engines. He knew the farm work trade and moved around from farm to farm living in tied cottages. When you took a job on a farm, a tied cottage usually went with it; finish the job and you were out of a home!

Samuel Jones, who died in 1965, was a severe, miserable man, but a genius with engines and he knew how to read and write – an uncommon thing in his generation. Children, however, in his eyes, were to be seen and not heard, and as grandchildren we never got close to him, and there were twenty-nine of us!

Grandmother Ellen, as I recall, was a large buxom lady who flowed around in long black skirts with a white pinafore around her ample waist. I do not remember much of her, as many of my childhood memories with her took place during my terrible illness. In later life, I visited her and my grandfather with my parents when she was very ill in bed with kidney failure. She was being nursed by various female members of the family, at Oakfields Farm near Hoarwithy.

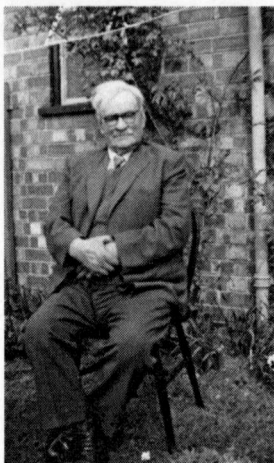

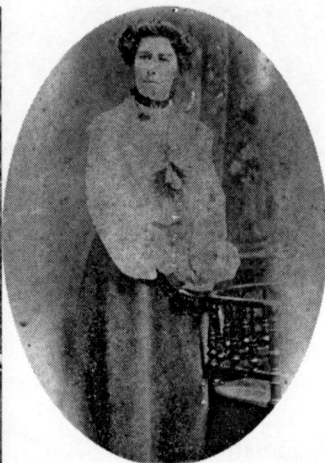

Granddad Samuel Jones in the 1950s; Grandmother Ellen Jones (née Gardiner)

During her illness, the district nurse used to call daily. She was a timid little spinster lady, one of a pair of twins, called Bessie. She was terrified of the dogs at Oakfields and would carry a whistle and use either the whistle or shout for aid before entering the high-stonewalled yard around the house.

Grandmother Jones died in 1951 when I was just ten years old. I can recall that it was my mother's turn to nurse her. We would stay over for a week at a time, or I would stay at home with Dad. One Saturday morning, I came down to find a huge pile of pillows on the stairs and landing. What was wrong? I knew something was, as there was a sort of hush around. Auntie Frances told me that Gran had died in the night; she was a very caring auntie, one of my favourites.

I asked where Granddad was and was told that he was fetching Mrs Lambe to lay out Grandmother. What was laying out? I have since learned that it is when a person dies and their body is put ready for the undertakers. This is what happened then; it is far different today!

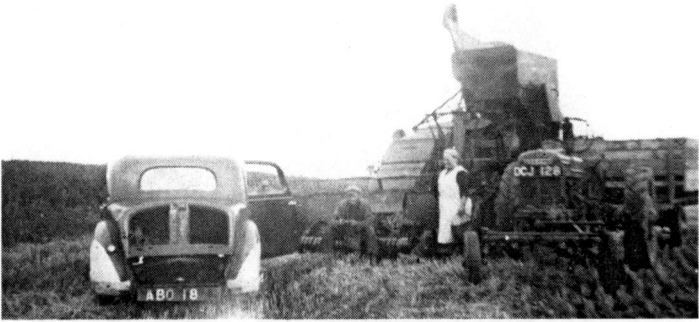

Grandmother Jones taking tea to the harvesters

When my grandfather and grandmother lived at Oakfields Farm, Hoarwithy, in the late 1940s and early 1950s (a tied house, which went with the job at Bromley Court, Hoarwithy), Gran would often be seen taking food to the men in the fields with her faithful basket. In the photograph is seen my grandmother, Ellen, Allan Gardiner (her nephew), and Gordon Roberts is sitting in the car with the registration number ABO18. Mr Roberts nicknamed this car the 'Always Buggering Off' car! The combine seen in the photograph is driven by the tractor in the front.

Eventually, my father, George Arthur Webb, and my mother, Clara Louisa Jones, were to meet at a dance at Brockhampton Village Hall. Dad was working at Chapel

Farm, How Caple, and my mother was by now working at Morney Cross, Fownhope, as a parlour maid.

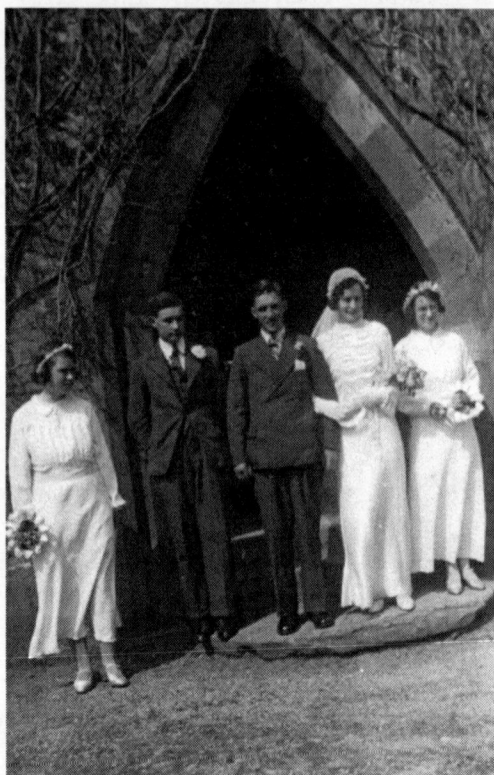

Wedding party outside Brockhampton Church, 18 April 1938

They were married at Brockhampton Church on 18 April 1938. Two of her sisters, Marjorie and Frances, were her bridesmaids, with Dad's best man being his cousin Leonard. My Grandfather Jones took a dislike to my dad, his prospective son-in-law, and threatened not to give my mother away at the ceremony. He took this attitude right up until the morning of the wedding, but just as my mother and

Lewis (her brother), who was to act as a stand-in father, were to leave for the church, he relented and drove with her in the car to the church. It is ironic that after the marriage my father and he were to become firm friends. There was a reception at the bride's home but no honeymoon. After the reception, the couple left for their new home at Lodge Cottage, Yatton.

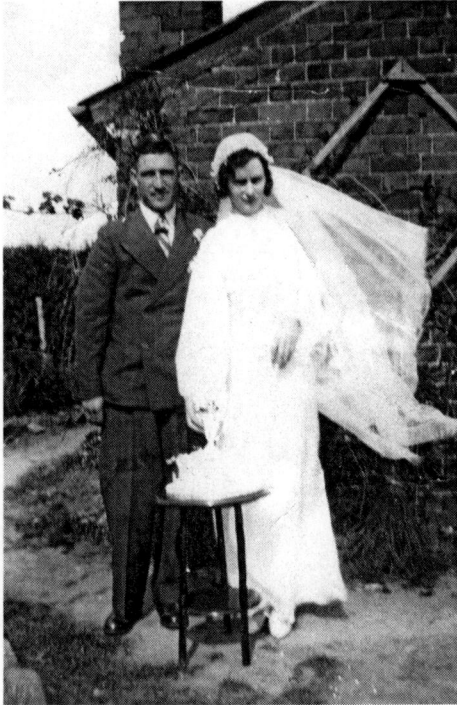

George and Clara Webb, cutting the cake

Lodge Cottage had no facilities, i.e. water and electricity, and no indoor toilet. George's job at Chapel Farm was a couple of fields' walk away.

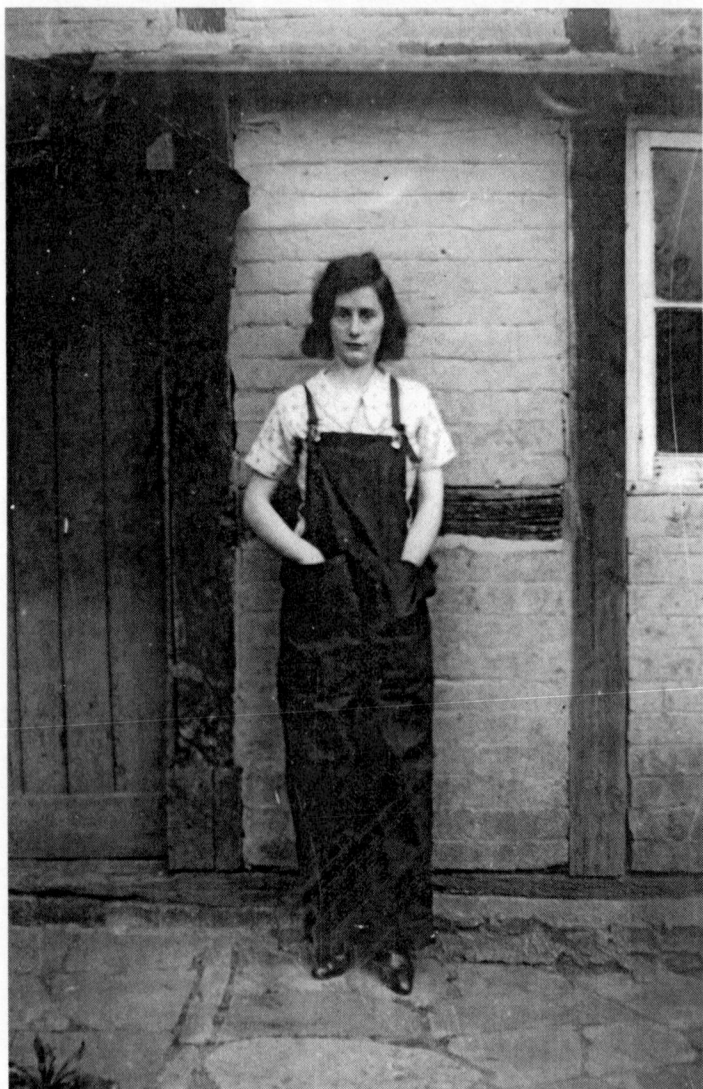

Clara at Lodge Cottage, Yatton

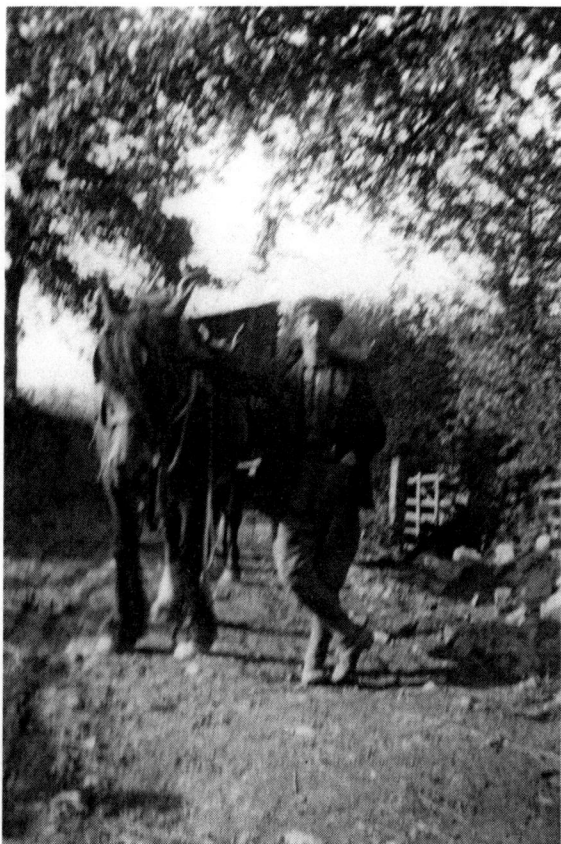

George outside Lodge Cottage with horse and cart

The couple did not stay there long, however, as they were offered a far superior cottage at How Caple, a small scattered village approximately halfway between the county town of Hereford and the small market town of Ross-on-Wye. This cottage was called Yew Tree Cottage. This was not a tied house, but rent was paid to the large Perrystone Estate. Wages from his agricultural work, tending the stock and doing arable work with horses, etc. amounted to £1 18s 6d per week (nearly £2 per week, £104 per annum), and the rent of the tiny cottage was 4s 6d per week.

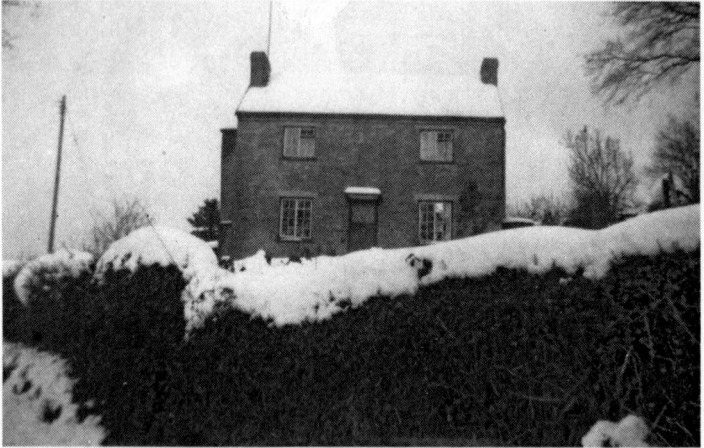

Yew Tree Cottage, How Caple, 1956

Yew Tree Cottage stood high on the hill at How Caple, and the view extended as far as the Black Mountains bordering Wales.

Chapter 2

Memories of my Early Years

Yew Tree Cottage is where I was born on 17 September 1941 at about 8 a.m. I was a bonny baby weighing in at a healthy 8 lb. The district nurse attended the birth. As she carried me downstairs to meet my dad, she said, 'This is Rosemary, your daughter.' To this, he said, 'Also add Elizabeth, after my mother, and she will be called Rosemary Elizabeth.'

In that year, 17 September fell on a Wednesday, and as the saying goes, 'Wednesday's child is full of woe'!

Ironically, during October of that year there was a big storm which blew some tiles from the roof. They were called 'Rosemary tiles'.

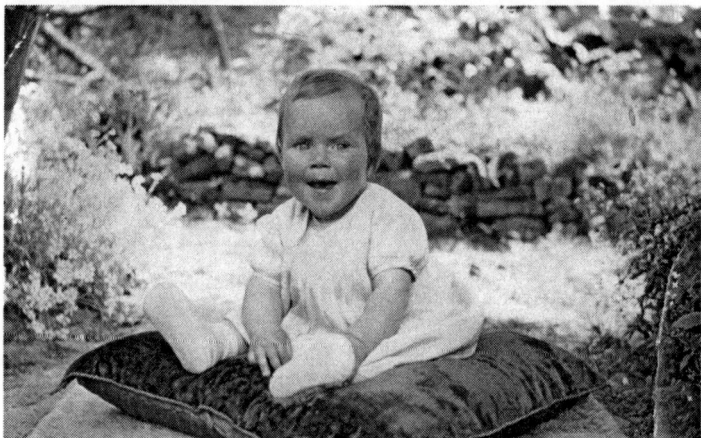

Author at nine months, Yew Tree Cottage

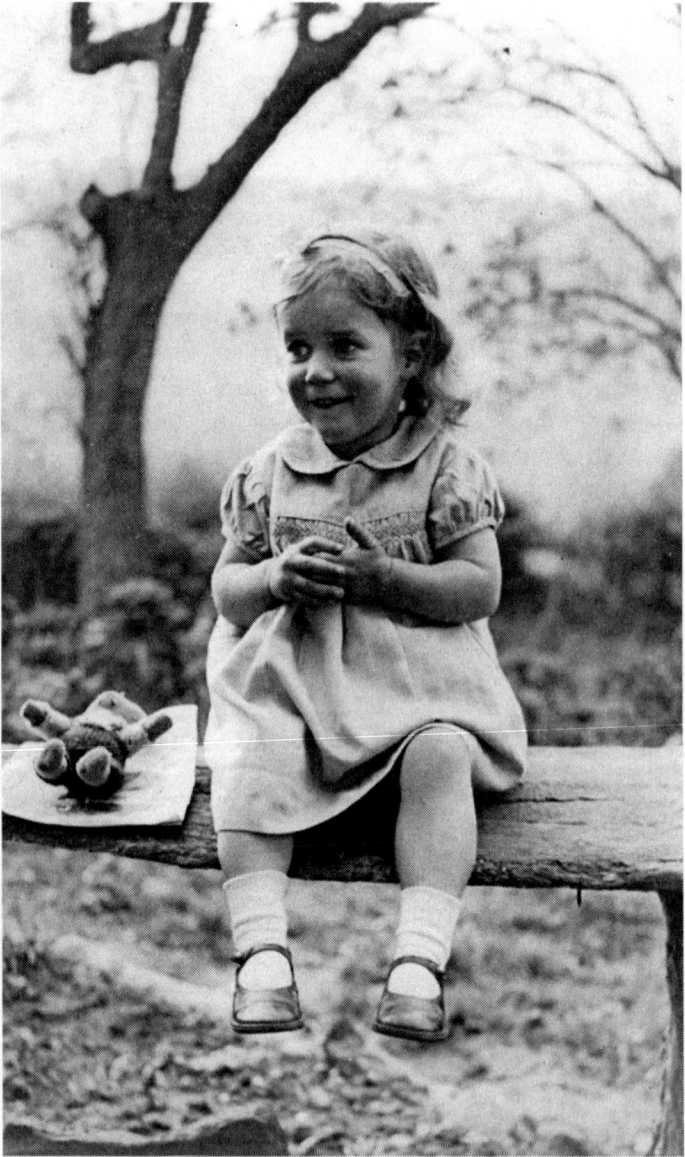
Author at two years, Yew Tree Cottage

Yew Tree Cottage was to be my home for the first 5½ to 6 years of my life. It was, and still is, a red-bricked detached house rebuilt from a thatched cottage burnt down in the 1930s, with two bedrooms, neither of which was bigger than about 14 ft square. There was a central staircase going up from the front door which ended on a landing, and each bedroom was reached by a further two steps. On this landing there was a small window which looked out onto the back of the house. I would stand on this landing and eagerly wait for my father to approach from his work at Chapel Farm, across the field. He and Fred Sollars from next door, at Ash Tree Cottage, were workmates at Chapel Farm and would walk home from work together. At the edge of the field they would part company, each going across the field to his own home. They both made their own personal path through whatever crop had been planted, usually wheat, oats or barley.

On the ground floor of Yew Tree Cottage there were two rooms corresponding in size to the bedrooms above. One was the front room, which we rarely used. In there was the best three-piece suite and a lovely mahogany round table. There was also an open fireplace, which had a fire in it at Christmas and high days and holidays. The other room was the living room. This was located across the tiny entrance hall and was only about 14 ft square. In here there was a blacklead cast-iron grate which was fuelled with wood and coal, with sway poles over it. The sway pole is the arm which carried the kettles and pots over the fire. We usually lived in this tiny room, where Dad had his old leather armchair, usually with a cat called Kitter sat on the arm. Mum had a more comfy chair, and I just sat on a stool or the settee or chaise longue. It must have been very cramped, as there were also a table and four chairs in this room! Off the living room was the pantry (under the stairs), and on the walls and over the fireplace hung sides of bacon, as Dad usually kept a pig in the cot in the garden.

Pig-killing day, which I hated, was awful. Our poor old pig was dragged out of his cot, squealing terribly, having had no supper, then was shot in the head and unceremoniously dragged onto a bench where his throat was cut. A fire of straw was lit and he (or she) was moved to the fire and burnt all over to get rid of the whiskers, then drenched in water and scrubbed all over with empty pilchard tins, which had holes punched in from the inside to make a sort of scrubbing tin. This done, the poor chap was dragged once again onto the pig bench where his insides were removed (i.e. heart, lungs, kidneys, etc.) and put into a tin bath. He was then hoisted upside down, attached to a beam in the back kitchen, for several days. Granddad Jones was the pig killer, who then proceeded to clean the guts in a bath of cold water with a hazel stick being pushed through the giblets. These were either used for sausages or salted and eaten as chitterlings. A few days later, the pig was cut up and the 'pig meat' (loin, in today's wording) distributed to anyone in and around, i.e. others who had pigs to kill and would return the favour. The rest – ham, shoulders, middle, etc. – would be salted with salt, salt petre and brown sugar on the salting stone in the back kitchen, usually slate and very heavy. This process took about three weeks. The salted meat was then hung up around the cottage in white cotton fly-proof bags and cut off and boiled or fried through the year.

As I have stated, the pig was salted on the salting stone which was housed in the back kitchen, which was attached to the back of the house. Also in this room there was a boiler with a fire underneath. This was used to heat the water to do the washing and also to have a bath (I will touch on washdays and bath days later in the story). Also in the back kitchen was the Primus stove and Primus stove cooker and oven. This was run on paraffin and methylated spirit.

Water for drinking was fetched in buckets from a well a quarter of mile away at the Pump Corner. Dad would set off with two buckets, with a yolk across his shoulders, to fetch the drinking water for the day. A yolk is a wooden framework shaped to fit the shoulders, with chain at each end on which to hang the buckets. Once at the Pump Corner, Dad would have to prime the well in order to get the pump started. On the adjacent side of the road was an open well, and usually there was a metal cup or mug or old tin with which people carried water from there to the pump in order to prime it. Once the water was poured down the pump's throat, the user had to pump furiously in order to get the water up, which then filled his two buckets. It was a lucky day if the person requiring water followed someone else who needed water. Then they would not have to prime the pump as well!

Dear Dad then set off home with his precious load, and once there he deposited it in the back kitchen on the top of the furnace, which had a wooden lid. This water was used only for drinking or cooking – nothing else. Beside the bucket there was usually a metal cup for ladling the water out with.

Now we come to washday. This involved a whole day's work. On the night before washday, Mother would have put the heavy clothes to soak in buckets. In the morning, she would wash the whites by hand and place them in the boiler, which she had previously filled with cold water and lit the fire underneath the boiler in order to get hot water. The precious two buckets of drinking water would have been placed in a place of safety while this procedure was going on. The whites would then be boiled for quite some time and then they were taken out with the aid of a pair of tongs, similar to those used in supermarkets today to take the cakes from the shelves. These tongs were, however, made of wood with a springy bit of metal holding the two arms together, and bleached white with continual dips in boiling water.

She would then put the whites in a bowl of soft water to rinse them, add a blue bag, which helped to make whites look whiter, and finally she would put them through the mangle. The same procedure followed for the remainder of the washing. It was all finally hung on the very long line to dry. There were no tumble driers then! It was a very hard day's work. Washing would dry very quickly as the line was across the garden facing the Black Mountains. Mum could see any storms coming and was able to get the washing in.

The water for washing, etc. was gathered from the roof of the tiny cottage into galvanised round tanks with a tap at the bottom. This was referred to as 'soft water', and it was marvellous to wash your hair in. It was indeed unfortunate if there was a long period of dry weather – no water!

Lastly came the ironing. Mum would have placed the washing on the long line across the top of the garden using the cane or wicker basket to carry it to and from the line. These baskets were usually made by blind people. Once back in the house, she would heat the flat irons (made of iron) in front of the open fire, on the lip of the grate. Flat irons had a handle and a flat base. There were usually thick home-made iron cloths used to pick up the flat irons from the grate. The iron, when hot, was picked up, wiped free of any smuts with another cloth, spat on to see if it was hot enough, and then off Mother went with her ironing.

Her ironing board consisted of several old, tatty blankets and a clean sheet on the top, quite thick in fact, and placed on the kitchen table. There were usually two or three irons on the go – one getting hot, or perhaps a bigger one for sheets, etc. Once all the ironing was done, she put the clean laundry on a clothes horse, a wooden contraption which folded down to a flat, portable affair. It usually had two or three portions. All was then placed in front of the fire to air in the winter, or outside in the sun in the summer and the clothes were then put away. The whole process then started again. Monday was usually washday, Tuesday ironing, Wednesday town, etc.

I haven't mentioned, so far, the bathroom and toilet. This property, along with many others in that era, had neither. The toilet was across the yard from the back door. Now this was my mother's pride and joy. It was housed in the last corrugated tin shed in a line of three; the others being used for coal and garden tools, and so on. In this little shed was a wooden seat with a large round hole cut into it, and under the seat there was a bucket with a lip facing the front, also a little wooden door with a catch on it, in order to get the bucket out. Our toilet was a one-seater with a bucket. My gran and granddad at Oakfields, Hoarwithy, had a three-seater – very grand! I did, in my childish mind, wonder why they had three seats – a large one, a medium one and a tiny one, the tiny one having a step. Did people go out to the toilets in parties? In my adult life I realised that when attending the toilet, usually on one's own, you chose the size of the hole you required! Dad used to get our bucket out from under the hole probably once a week. To be honest, I don't know how many times it was emptied.

Gran and Granddad's toilet was an earth closet. The human waste just dropped into a pit and the flies and nature got rid of it. This establishment was quite a way from the house, obviously because of the smell, so it was a long trek from the house to the toilet in the dark.

My Auntie Frances (my mother's sister) at Oakfields would carry a candle in a jam jar and remark, 'Just going down south, won't be long!' If you didn't go before going to bed, you would resort to using a chamber pot – one under each bed, a 'goesunder'!

By the seat at either our house toilet or at Gran's house

there would be toilet paper, usually Izal, a brand of strong medicated toilet paper, or newspaper cut up into little squares. Those little squares of toilet paper would usually be read more than the paper it originally came from.

On washdays, my mother would carry a bucket of hot soapy water across the yard and give the seat a good scrub. This was a bit unfortunate if you were in a hurry, because the seat took a long time to dry and you could end up with quite a damp bottom!

All around this lovely cottage, set into the bank of a field, was a lovely cottage garden. Mum would tend the flowers and Dad would tend his veggies when he returned from the farming duties at night. He always emptied the toilet bucket into a hole in the garden which had previously been dug, so no wonder cottage gardens to this day produce such lovely vegetables. The bucket was never carried very far and the hole was always dug in advance, as no one lingered on this job! It was always Dad's job; I never remember Mum emptying the bucket, unless in dire emergencies, such as when Dad was ill.

The smell of the lovely flowers from our garden are always strong in my memory – the 'Mrs Sinkins' pinks, the white lilies and the lilac in the spring. At the front of the cottage were yew tree stumps, where two yew trees had once stood. It was where the cottage got its name from. In later years, my dad and Uncle Fred (from next door) spent a whole evening sawing these two stumps off with a cross-cut saw. Cross-cut saws are very big and require two men to operate. They have hundreds of razor-sharp teeth. Yew is a very, very hard wood, and I can remember spending the whole evening pouring water on the saw to keep it cool.

The cottage and garden were very much open to the elements, and the rain and wind would lash in from the Welsh hills over thirty miles away. I am still nervous of the wind to this day. I cannot feel safe with it. I remember persuading my dad to move my bed away from the window in case the wind blew me out of my bed!

In those days snow was also a problem, in that it usually filled our little lane up. I vaguely remember the great snow of 1947 and the blizzard which started on 4 March, when we could not get out and could not see the cottage next door. That tiny little cottage, also tucked into the bank, disappeared into a giant snowdrift. I apparently said to my mother that we would not see Uncle Fred and Aunt Edith's cottage in the morning and, lo and behold, come the morning we couldn't!

As mentioned before, we did not have a bathroom or water at Yew Tree Cottage. A daily wash was obtained by boiling a kettle over the fire and mixing this with cold water until the required temperature was obtained. With flannel and towel in hand, you proceeded to wash in the back kitchen, with little privacy and no heat!

Every weekend we all had a bath. Mother would, once again, light a fire under the furnace and load it with soft water from the outside tanks. She would also place, near the bath, a couple of buckets of cold soft water, for mixing! Bathing was by way of a six-foot-long tin bath, which, when not in use, was hung on a peg by the back door. I was the first into the bath, then Mum and finally Dad. It must have been fairly grotty by the end, but Dad, being a polite man, never grumbled. This procedure was OK in summer, but in the winter the only heat was from the little furnace door which Mum would open – but the door was only about twelve inches square!

Once bathed, it was a quick towel down, as you did not linger in the cold, and then, once you were dressed, usually in nightclothes for us all, the bath was dragged outside and tipped out, either on the vegetable patch or left to run down the storm drain. Hair-washing was not done as frequently as it is these days. The water for that would be heated by a kettle over the fire and mixed with some cold water. You would dip your head in and Mum would rub in some shampoo and rub like mad. Some additional water, which had been prepared to the correct temperature, was poured on by cup to rinse the hair. It was a lengthy and miserable experience!

Heating the house was done by way of an open range in the living room, an open fire in the sitting room, and a little weeny fireplace in each bedroom. The bedroom fireplaces were only lit if someone was ill. The wood and the coal would be hauled in from the shed. Dad would bring home wood from the orchards at Chapel Farm from trees felled by storms and chop it into logs.

All cooking was done on the open range by way of a sway pole over the fire or on the paraffin stove (Primus) in the back kitchen, but how it worked I don't quite remember. Soups and stews seemed to be continually produced from the range, the most popular being chicken and vegetable. The range was blacklead, and Mum spent many hours polishing it with Zebo, getting very black hands in the process, and of course there were no rubber gloves in those days.

Lighting was supplied by several oil lamps and candles, the oil having been delivered by George Nicholls of Ross-on-Wye, who was a hardware merchant, carrying everything in a little van, including the oil, which was dispensed into our own metal, two-gallon can from a tank in the back of the van. In the winter months, Mother would trim and fill up the oil lamps ready for night. There was always a lamp in the living room. When I was a little older, progress was made in that Dad purchased a Tilley lamp. This was a wonderful new light which worked on pressure, and once the light began to fade, furious pumping took place and the light gradually got brighter and brighter. This was a wonderful new invention. Going to bed was a difficult procedure, in that you had a candle each in an old metal candlestick. These were considered safer than the taller ornamental variety.

An electricity pole was placed in the garden near the cottage by the landlords, the Perrystone Estate, and later on, in June 1949, electricity arrived in the house. Mum and Dad had been so desperate to improve their living accommodation that they had made enquiries and said they themselves would pay for the electricity to be installed. The cost would be £49. The Midlands Electricity man came and put one plug and one light socket in each room. I remember the man saying that one should not take wet to electricity as they do not mix, and this is a fact I remember to this day. Mum and Dad purchased a little Belling electric hob and oven, and new saucepans to go with it. My mother used those saucepans until her death in early 2008! The wonderful new bright light was exciting, with just a switch to control it – but a bill to pay each quarter.

We still continued to listen each evening to the wireless, which was powered by batteries. There was a 'dry' battery (high tension) which would last about eight to ten weeks and one accumulator battery. The accumulator battery accompanied the dry battery which ran the radio. Users had two accumulator batteries, one for use and one away being charged. The man who charged the batteries lived in Yatton, about a mile and a half's walk away through the dark and spooky Yatton Woods – not a trip for the faint-hearted! Dad would walk winter and summer through the woods, and in later years I would accompany him in order to see my godmother, Alice Sollars, and her husband, Uncle Jim, and my good friend, their daughter, Maureen.

Dick Barton was on the radio in those days and I was an avid fan. Dick, Snowy and Jock joined us in our living room each night. We were also joined by *PC49*, a half-hour comedy programme about a hapless police constable. Mum was not a fan of *Dick Barton*, and when this was on she would just sit and do her knitting.

The postman delivered a paper each day, rolled up with our address written on a piece of paper wrapped around the middle. Dad enjoyed the paper, but was never keen on the crossword. Mum, however, did enjoy the crossword and always enjoyed the letters page.

Dad was not highly paid as an agricultural worker, but he was surprised and delighted one day to be presented with a Fordson tractor, for use on Chapel Farm. This replaced his horses, and he soon got into the ways of using his new toy and of having to turn it off to go to lunch!

Dad would supplement his income in the autumn by going cider-apple picking in the orchards at Chapel Farm for about one shilling a hessian bag (5p). He would take the faithful Tilley lamp to see by at night. He worked very hard and tried hard to save a little for those luxuries in life. Up until the time we had electricity, we must have had two Tilley lamps – one for home and one for Dad to work at night by.

Dad would also go blackberry picking in the autumn. Chapel Farm nestled into the hillside at How Caple, with steep rough banks rising above the farmyard. On those rough banks grew copious amounts of blackberry bushes. They were very dense bushes, as no machines or horses could get there to mow. Dad and Mum, if she was out picking too, would have to tread down the surrounding area to reach the larger fruits on the tops of the bushes. In later years I recall seeing many snakes, both adders and grass snakes, sunning themselves on Snowy Hill, or creeping along near to the wet area in the Dark Orchard. Dad, however, seemed oblivious to the danger of snakes and he went picking well into the autumn nights; how he ever saw the little black fruit in the shadowy light was a mystery to me.

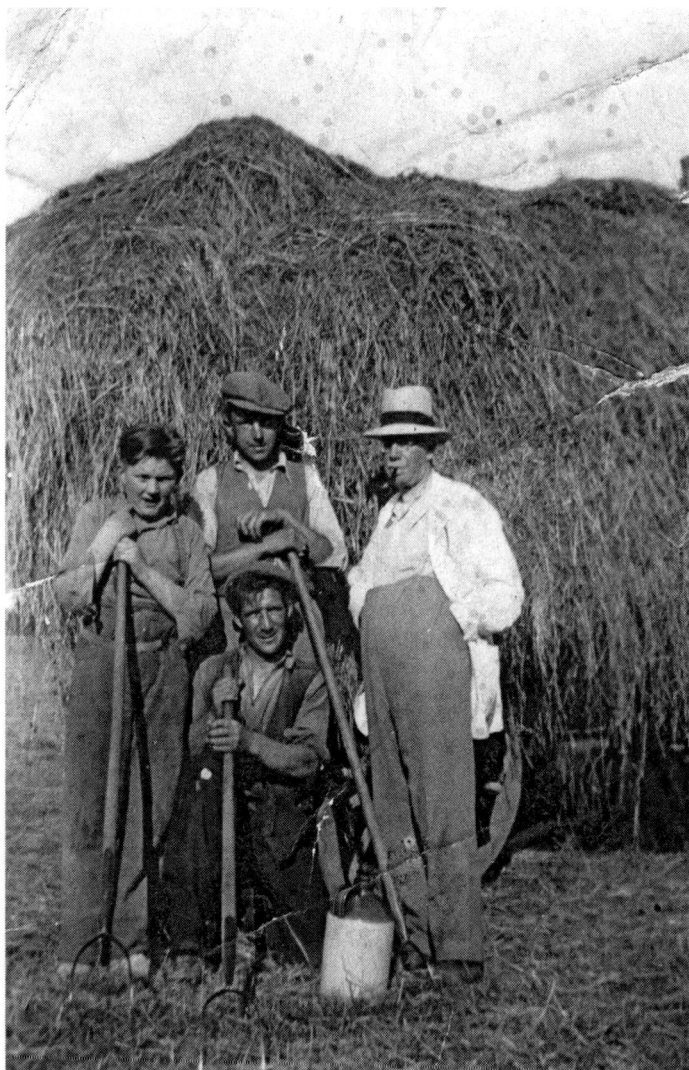

Haymaking
Left to right: John Ford, Harry Ford, Staunton Calvert (Dad's boss's father)
Front: George Webb

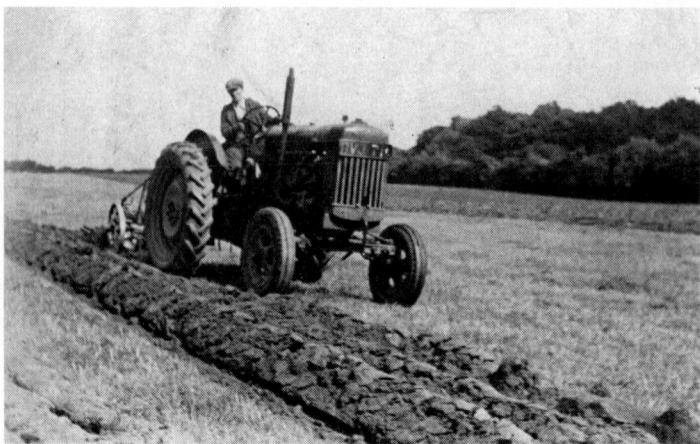

George with his tractor and plough

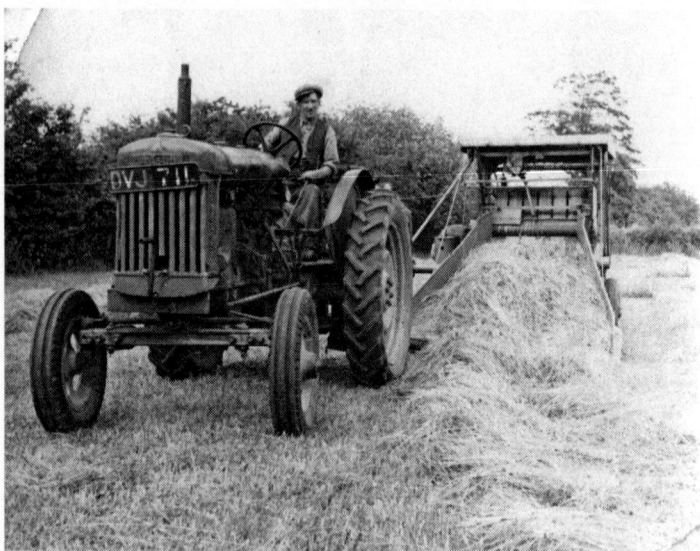

George with a round baler (little round bales, like sausages!)

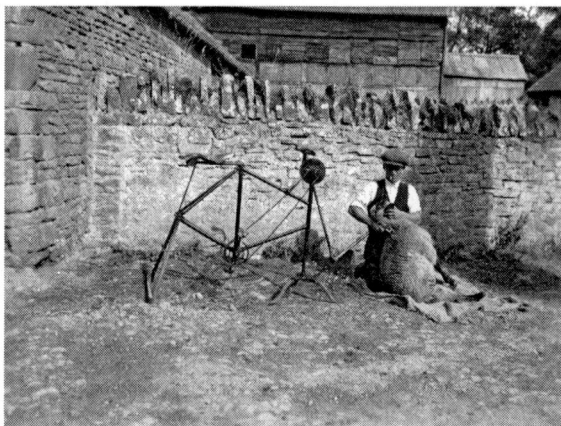

George Webb, shearing

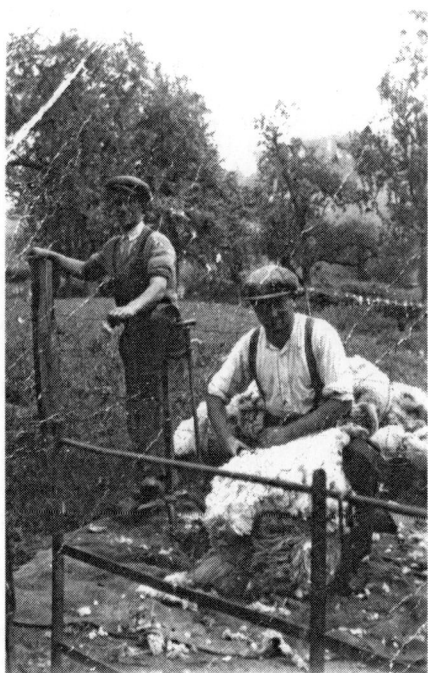

Blackberry income was very valuable in those days. All types of receptacles were used, from buckets to baths and washing-up bowls – in fact, anything you could find to accommodate the little black fruit as, on a Tuesday and a Thursday, Mr Brown from Ross and his little red lorry would call, weigh your fruit and pay you. Mr W J Brown's advertisement read:

WANTED – TONS OF BLACKBERRIES DAILY.
TELEPHONE ROSS-ON-WYE 2069.

This was good money, which was duly put away. Usually, it was about 3d a pound, I believe, but it would vary from week to week. All receptacles empty, Dad and Mum would start the process all over again, ready for Mr Brown next week. The blackberries were sent away in large containers to factories to make dye. That is what we believed them to be used for, because if they were used for jam or jelly they would have been very mouldy, having been picked for several days. Mr Brown, whose hands were very stained from the blackberries, was also a dealer in country products and would pay for rabbits, hens, apples and mushrooms in the autumn, or indeed anything he could sell on.

Dad enjoyed hedge-laying and would spend many a Saturday in winter and early spring at a hedging match. He once came home with the coveted Cup, much to the annoyance of the acclaimed champion, who moaned and groaned that he'd had a bad length, and my dad had had a good one, that's why he'd won. What a bad loser!

Hedge-laying is a traditional method of controlling a hedge when it has grown too high. The hedge is then laid. You start with a chain length (which, in a hedging match, is 22 yards) and about 12 ft high or so, sort out the bushes and rough bits, and usually you are left with hawthorn, nut or other material standing about 6–12 inches apart, unless of course the hedge is dead in that section. It is advisable to wear big leather mittens – i.e. the fingers in one large section and the thumb in another, as the thorns of the blackthorn are lethal and will poison the system if entry is made into the skin. The equipment needed is an axe, a hacker and a mallet.

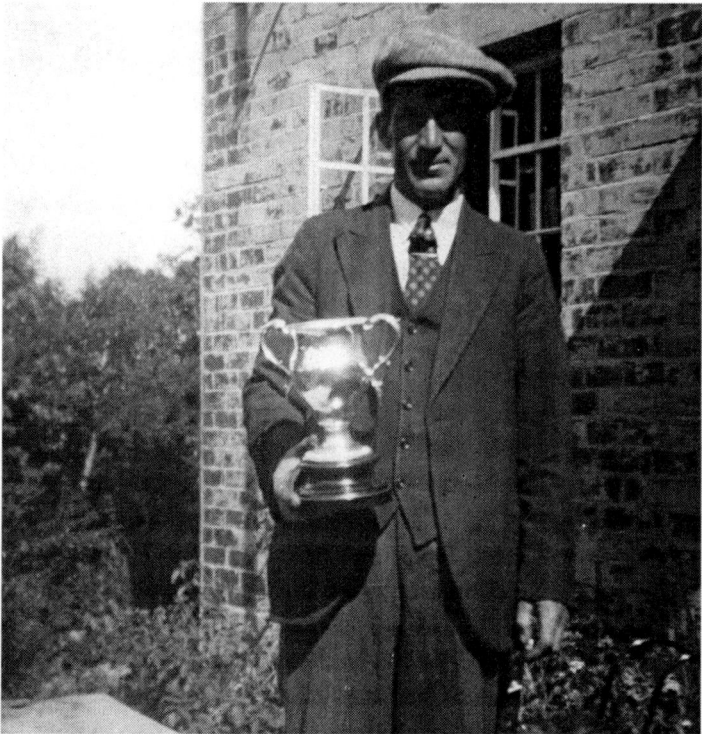

George with his Champion's Cup – a proud man
Yew Tree Cottage

Today's hedge-layers use chainsaws and the like. Stakes which had previously been cut were driven into the ground at regular intervals along the line of the hedge, at an angle, which was governed by the lie of the land, ditches, water-courses, and so on, or the boundaries. The next process is difficult to describe in writing, but using a hacker (or an axe if the pleacher is too big), a cut or incision is made in a downward fashion about 6–8 inches above ground level in the pleacher. Now, a pleacher is the material still standing up after you have done your first sort out. The cut is made in the pleacher just deep enough for it to be lain down without it snapping – an art which is acquired with experience. Once the pleacher is pliable enough to be laid down, it is gently eased down, weaving it in and out of the driven stakes. Then it is pressed down. This procedure is repeated, using odds and ends of pulled-out material if the hedge looks too thin at the end of the day. Hedge-laying for a living and not for a match took many days, and usually stopped once the leaves on the hedge started to show in spring.

The final part of hedge-laying is the driving home of the stakes and putting on the heatherings. These are long, slender and pliable pieces of hazel which are woven in and out of the stakes – usually two pieces, one on each side, forming a sort of plait. To make it look absolutely neat, the hacker or hedge bill is used to trim the sides of the hedge, and at a hedging competition the ditch on one side had to be dug out for a completed job. Hedging matches without the ditching are still held today. In those days, a competitor had to complete a chain of hedging and ditching in a day. I don't know how many yards (or metres) competitors do today.

In the spring, Dad and Uncle Fred[*] would do overtime at the farm. This consisted mostly of root-hoeing for mangolds, swedes, turnips and sugar beet. I remember one fateful day when there was a thunderstorm in the late evening and Dad and Uncle Fred had to retire from root-

---

[*] I had many adopted 'uncles', such as Uncle Fred and Uncle Jim.

hoeing on Barrel Hill. How Caple soil is very sandy, and when they went back the next day the whole crop had been washed into the road.

Dad worked very hard to support both Mum and me and put a little money away for luxuries. Mum also had a little job. She went to 'do' for Mrs Gordon across the road at the big house called 'The Cross'. She went on Tuesday and Friday mornings, and did general things like vacuuming and polishing. Mrs Gordon had the luxury of a vacuum cleaner. She was a very nice lady, who was divorced and had one daughter, Biddy, who lived away in Italy. Mrs Gordon had a companion called Miss Foster, who was a real old maid, but likeable with it. How much my mother earned I do not know, but she worked very hard. Real coffee (not Camp, which was out of a bottle and had chicory essence added to it) was taken at 10.30 a.m. I can still hear Mrs Gordon calling, 'Coffee, Mrs Webb, when you're ready!'

My memories of Yew Tree Cottage are happy ones. I understand that there is a point in your life where you start to remember your younger days more clearly and I remember many things from when I was only five or six.

I was happy but a little lonely. I had few friends my own age, save for Phillip Sollars, who lived next door, and my godmother's daughter, Maureen. I didn't see her very often as she lived quite a walk away. I did, of course, see a lot of Phillip, and we would chat over the garden fence. Phillip was much older than me, and he had the nickname Tchaikovsky or 'Tchaik' for short, after the composer. To this day I do not know why he was called this. He was a very clever lad, and later went on to Grammar School. Derek, his brother, was much younger than me, being born during the snowy period in early 1947. He does not feature at all in my story. The only thing I remember was that he was nicknamed 'Nutch' in later years as he was mad about Nuffield tractors, but could only say 'Nutchfield'.

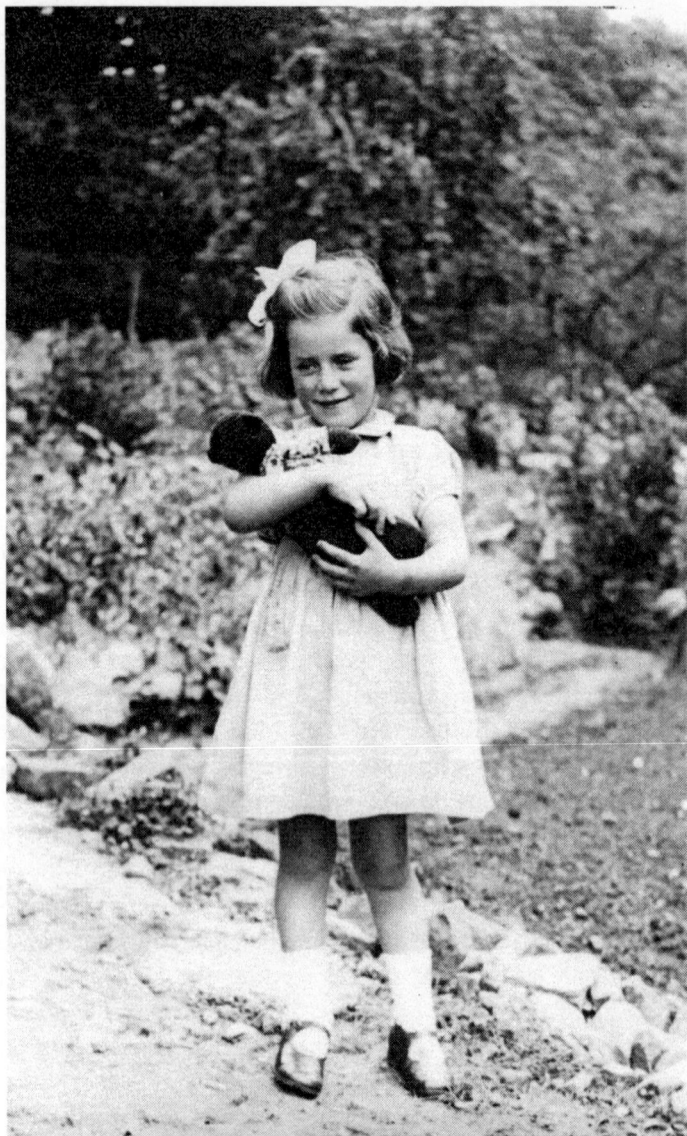

Author at four years old
Yew Tree Cottage

Chapter 3

Starting School

I started school in the autumn term of 1946 when I was just five years old. The primary school I attended was How Caple Primary School, which was just about quarter of a mile away. This was a two-room school with high ceilings and a pot-bellied solid fuel stove in the corner of each room which was fuelled with coke. The pot-bellied stoves, which gave out tremendous heat, were put into action if your coat and shoes got wet. All items were placed around the stoves on the guards and the steam would gently rise, just like a Chinese laundry. If anyone was ever poorly, they would be placed by the stove on a chair and minded, as usually parents would not be at home, and in any case the teacher could not leave the school to take you home. These two rooms were made out of one room which was partitioned. If you ever needed one room, the partition wall was concertinaed back across and one room was created. I never did see this done, but I believe it was done for social activities such as dances or whist drives. We used to write on slates using chalk and did not use pencils and paper.

The school was attached to the head teacher's house. Our head teacher was Mrs Nora Watkins, and she and her husband lived in the head teacher's house, which we walked sedately by each morning and evening to arrive at or leave the school.

Also attached was a piece of very muddy land and a garden which sloped down to the main road. The muddy land was affectionately known as 'The Playground'. It appeared huge to me in those days, and was in fact a bare piece of ground. We did PE out there and also took our playtime outside when it wasn't raining.

Our PE consisted of running on the spot, arms raised, then out, in, etc., etc. Winter or summer, we did this morning ritual and usually wore our navy-blue knickers, as we did not have the right kit, and changed into our navy-blue 'daps'. These were a sort of canvas shoe. I believe they are still worn in schools today.

Also at playtime we would drink our third of a pint of milk, which we loved, although it was 'raw' milk, not pasteurised. It came in a little bottle ($^1/_3$ pint) and we drank it through a straw. Sometimes in the winter the milk would be frozen, having been left waiting in the sub-zero temperatures outside the door for hours, or sour if it was left out in the sun in the summer! Milk was to play a big part in my life, as you will see over the following chapters.

We played cricket and rounders and all the other childhood games such as skipping and hopscotch. Other than that we just chatted, as children do. Up some steps from the playground were the toilets, girls on the left and boys on the right. These, again, were bucket toilets with a seat, which Mr Watkins (the head teacher's husband) would empty weekly. There was no luxury of flush toilets. If nature called, you would put your hand up, get your coat and go. When returning, you washed your hands in cold water in the cloakroom before returning to the classroom.

When I started, my teacher was Mrs Avery; she was the reception teacher. I enjoyed this new experience. We sat side by side with another pupil at all-in-one desks and seats. After we had had PE every morning, and when we arrived in class, we would say the Lord's Prayer, the Ten Commandments and the twelve times tables. It always came out parrot-fashion, but has held me in good stead these sixty-odd years. I can still repeat the twelve times tables, much to the amazement of my grandchildren.

Mrs Avery was an old woman, to my way of thinking. She would walk to school up the main road from her home at How Caple crossroads, oblivious to the occasional (and it was occasional in the 1940s) passing car, which would swerve around the old lady. It's a wonder she didn't get run over. Every afternoon she would tell us a story, but usually she fell asleep halfway through! We would watch as her head slowly fell lower are lower until she was sound asleep and often snoring. We never misbehaved, though, as Mrs Watkins was next door and at the sound of any mischief she would be through the door to us. I do remember, however, one day Kenny and Bobby Francis, Tony Hope and a couple of other lads decided to play a trick on the old lady. They quietly used a ruler to push the clock forward one hour, and when she awoke she mistakenly assumed that it was time to go home. We were all told we could go! I don't remember the outcome of this little adventure. Did we all get home an hour early, or did we enjoy a game or two in the lanes on the way home?

Pupils didn't wear uniforms in the 1940s or even 1950s. I remember being dressed in a home-made stripy jersey and a navy-blue pinafore dress with short white socks. Mum always insisted on my wearing a liberty bodice, which is a form of vest which buttoned down the front. I hated it and it tickled, as it was made of wool. Other underwear consisted of navy-blue knickers. Shoes had to be of a sensible design. My hair was always neatly combed with a ribbon in it.

Yew Tree Cottage was a stone's throw from the village school, and as it was down a country road, which was very quiet and with no danger from traffic, we usually walked in the middle of the road. In the early days, my mother would walk me down to school. After leaving the cottage, we walked down the garden path to the road, and then turned right. A little further on there was a gateway leading to a very narrow lane, which was at the end of Mrs Gordon's garden. It was quite a sloping walk to the school. I usually ran all the way down the narrow lane, which had hedges on either side, sliding to a halt when reaching the large kissing gate at the bottom. The lane had secret nooks and crannies all the way down. On the right, about halfway down, was the kitchen garden belonging to the big house where Mum worked. Bill Allsop was the head gardener there, and always grew lovely strawberries. If we were lucky, we were sometimes given some.

I never did it, but the boys would scrump apples and plums from the garden. They were always on a safe bet, as Bill could not run, as he had two artificial legs which squeaked as he walked with the aid of two sticks. It was a bit unfair, really, for the boys to do this to this kind old man just because they knew he couldn't chase them! He was a marvellous man because he always dug and cultivated the garden with no machinery at all. Our imaginations ran wild as we imagined Mr Allsop with no legs. He lost his legs in railway accident; he must have been a very brave man to carry on with his gardening.

How Caple School catchment area not only served the children of the small scattered village and parish of How Caple but also took pupils from the surrounding areas of Sollershope, Yatton and some from Foy to the east. My friends from Sollershope, Topsy (real name Rosemary), her sister, Joy, and their two brothers, John and Phillip, would walk to school, as did most of the pupils. They would form a 'walking bus', picking up the Hope boys on the way – Tony, Bill and Vernon, who were the youngest children of a family of thirteen. They, in turn, would pick up the Francis boys, Kenny and Bobby.

There were no thoughts in these days of anything happening to any of us. There were always people around who knew who you were and looked out for you. The roadmen (lengthmen) looked after the roads, each man having a set length of road. He would be in full control of his 'length', seeing to the ditches, gullies, drains, etc. and would very often chat to whomever came by, either by foot or in a car or on a bicycle. Our 'lengthman' was George Kempshaw, a stern old man who lived in a cottage around towards Yatton.

The farm workers always knew who you were and we always felt safe walking in the countryside. At dinner time, if you lived close by, you went home to dinner. Those pupils who did not live close to the school had school dinners out of dreadful pale stainless-steel or enamel containers. The custard and gravy looked awful, and sure enough it was awful, all lumpy and thick. The dinners would arrive late morning in a little blue van. They then just sat there until dinner time, when Mrs Watkins and Mrs Avery donned their checked aprons and served the dinners. I sometimes had dinner at school and sometimes went home to lunch, depending on whether or not my parents were at home.

Dinners were taken in the classroom. Two tables were unfolded from against the wall and laid out with chairs, which were stacked. We couldn't use our desks, as they were all-in-one seat and desk, with inkwells in each right-hand corner. Ink was made up by the ink monitor from a black powder and water and was taken around by the monitor about once a week.

Chapter 4
Telling my Story

The next couple, or maybe three, years of my young life were suddenly to alter in a very dramatic way.

I suppose for the last sixty-odd years I have kept memories stored in my memory bank and not aired them to the world at large. Then I went to a meeting of the local WI one winter's night towards the end of the twentieth century. The local radio station was looking for people to tell their story in a broadcast called 'The Century Speaks'. To cut a long story short, I contacted the radio station and they were indeed interested in what I am about to relate to readers. Along with my late mother, Mrs Clara Webb, I was interviewed for the programme, and snippets of the interview were broadcast.

The interviewer also took me by car to Nieuport Sanatorium (with the present owner's permission) to look around. I am undecided whether this was a good thing or a bad, but certainly on looking at 'my room' shivers went down my back. I have also, with my husband, been back to Jan Smuts Home, which is now an old people's home. They were thrilled to show me around and I had a photo enlarged and framed for them.* They were delighted with it and marvelled at the dresses of the sisters in the picture.

Ever since that broadcast, I have wanted to put down my memories of that dreadful period in my life, but I hesitated. I have, however, succeeded, and in the next few chapters I will try to portray to readers the dreadful conditions in

_____
* As seen on page 108

hospitals in the 1940s; my mother's and father's anguish at finding out that their only daughter was about to die; the sometimes tender, loving care of the staff at hospitals, and the sometimes uncaring attitude of other staff. I shall also try to capture the stand-offish behaviour of neighbours and so-called friends when they realised I had a contagious disease, i.e. tuberculosis, and how I felt like a leper in their midst. I also feel that these facts should be put down so that future generations can read about life in hospitals in the 1940s, and how very, very different it was from today.

Chapter 5

Falling Ill and the Holiday

I had always felt comfortable and happy in my home at Yew Tree Cottage. The only time I ever felt frightened there was when it was windy, but generally it had a lovely atmosphere.

When did I first start to feel ill? It was in the spring of 1947, the first term of the year at school and my second term of attendance. During the April I developed whooping cough, a bad illness for children. I remember coughing a lot. It is a very exhausting illness. This illness usually only lasts a few weeks, but my coughing and general ill health went on and on. I wouldn't have realised it, but I was losing weight and had become very pale in complexion. My curly hair no longer had its lustre and I was generally under the weather. I had very blonde curly hair as a child, which people would often remark about.

How ill was I? Children do not ask these questions. I still had a dreadful cough and it was going on and on. Home visits were made by the family doctor, Dr Godfrey Malkin. He was a kindly old man, to my eyes, always gentle and caring. How was medical aid paid for before the NHS? My mother told me she paid into a sort of private healthcare system. I don't know much about it.

Dr Malkin's surgery was in Fownhope, about four miles towards Hereford. As I have said, he was a lovely old gentleman, and a good GP. His surgery was antiquated and small, as was the waiting room. There was no appointments system, surgery usually starting at 9 a.m. till 11 a.m. in the morning and after home visits 6 p.m. till 7 p.m. in the evening.

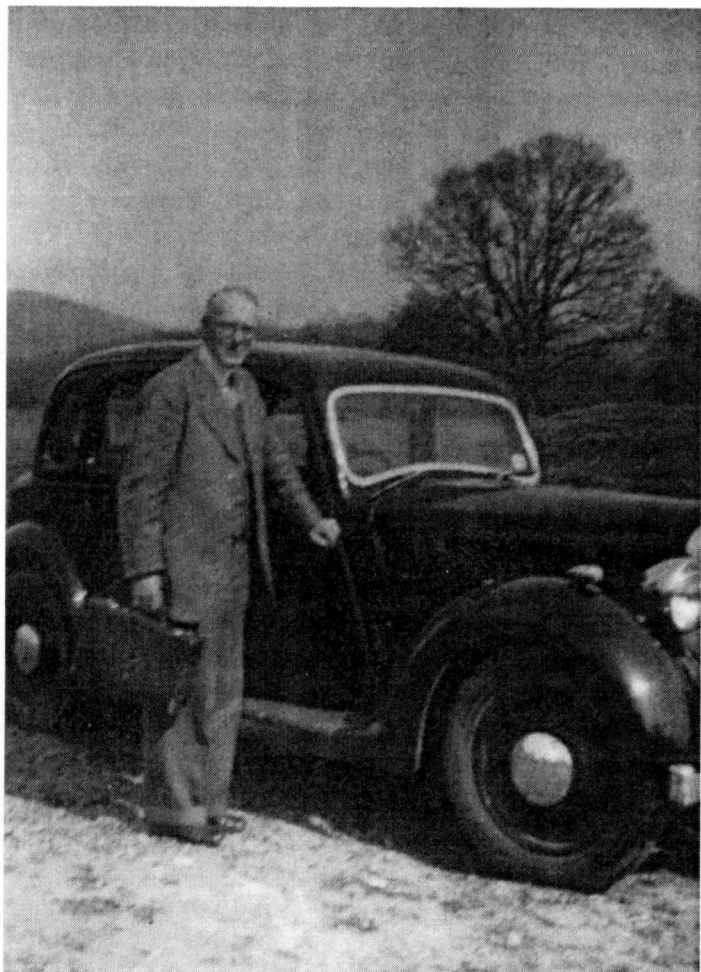

Dr G Malkin beside his car in 1953
Image reprinted courtesy of Mrs N Cope

Patients attended and sat in the waiting room on the long bench and Dr Malkin would put his head round the door and say 'Next, please.' When the first patient in line moved into the doctor's surgery, the next person moved up one seat, and so on. You then entered his tiny domain, which housed his huge desk, plus a filing cabinet with all his patients' notes, a small dispensary, a fold-down couch and two chairs (one for him and one for the patient).

My notes were always next to those of a girl named Rosanna Webb, and there was often some confusion when the doctor pulled her notes out instead of mine. The walls of Dr Malkin's office, like those of the waiting room, were covered in shelves and shelves of medicine in large bottles. Colours ranged from pink, to green and red. When you had told the doctor your problem and he had made a diagnosis, he then proceeded to make up the cure, whether it was tablets or medicine.

His surgery finished when the last patient went home, which could be ten o'clock at night. Dr Malkin had a car to do his rounds and if he was out at night, his wife would put a light on on the landing to tell the doctor not to put the car away if he was required to go out again.

Home visits were the norm, then, and his stethoscope was always very cold. There was no central heating, of course, and so I undressed in front of the fire, where Dr Malkin examined me. It was just after a spell of horren-dous weather and the whole house was chilly. Dr Malkin was wearing his smart pinstripe suit and he smelt of carbolic. All the people around me had serious but smiling faces. How had I contracted whooping cough, and why was it not clearing up as it should do? Something was very wrong…

During one of those spring mornings, my mother has since told me, I had a turn and went blue. Dad hurried across to Mrs Gordon's (the only person with a phone) and telephoned Dr Malkin, who came more or less immediately. He examined me with that dreadfully cold stethoscope. My colour had apparently returned to normal by then and he suspected asthma. He asked a lot of questions as to whether there was a history of asthma in the family. A few weeks passed, and by this time I was *very* thin and not eating. Nothing would tempt me; I just would not eat! Dr Malkin now suggested X-rays and a hospital visit was arranged, with an appointment to see a specialist, a Dr Phillip.* By this time it was July 1947.

One day, Mum and I set off on the bus, the dear old Midland Red bus which passed through How Caple on the main road between Hereford and Ross-on-Wye. If you were going to Ross, you boarded the bus at Cross-in-Hands because it was cheaper, and if you were going to Hereford you would board at How Caple Crossroads for the same reason. Both stops were about a mile apart. We did not own a car at the time, although Dad had a driving licence. I suppose we couldn't afford one. Mr Calvert, Dad's employer at Chapel Farm, had a car, a large Austin. He could well afford a car as he was what is called a 'gentleman farmer'. He bought a new one very frequently. Mrs Gordon also owned a car; sometimes she would drive and sometimes she would be chauffeured. Her car was a black Morris Oxford.

The appointment for X-rays was at the General Hospital in Hereford, the same hospital where my grandfather had died of his injuries in 1912. In those days there was a waiting time for the X-rays to be developed. An appointment was made to see a specialist that day – Dr Phillip – who would discuss the result of the X-rays later, when they were developed. My mum was told not to worry unduly by Dr Phillip, but he suggested that perhaps a little holiday

---

* Dr Phillip was a specialist in lung disorders at the County Hospital.

would do us good. Coincidentally, Mum had already arranged a holiday. Just my mother and I were to take this two-week holiday, as Dad did not have many holidays from his farm work and he was more than capable of fending for himself at home. Mum had decided that we should go to her brother-in-law and her sister Gladys's little farm, which nestled under the Black Mountains near Longtown, Herefordshire. This little rented farm was called The Kellyn, and I loved going there as I met up with my cousins, Irene, who was a nurse, and Percy, who was at Lady Hawkins' School in Kington.

Gran and Granddad offered to take Mum and me to The Kellyn in their little Austin motor car.

The Kellyn is perched high on a hill looking across the valley to the first range of the Black Mountains and the Cat's Back next to the first range of Black Mountains. The Cat's Back is called this as it is said that it is so narrow to walk along that it is like walking on a thin cat's back. Here, as at Yew Tree Cottage, the weather would throw itself at the house throughout most of the winter. The house was stone built, with four windows facing the mountains. The windows were glazed with lead and glass, and I'm sure that every one of those little diamonds let the rain in. The house did not have central heating, so each of the rooms had a little fireplace in it. Depending on which room Uncle Cecil and Auntie Gladys were living in, there was usually a great big fire going in the winter. The floor had gigantic grey flagstones set together, and on these there were several hand-made pulled-rag mats tossed casually about.

There was a central passage which had no natural light and out of this there was a huge stone step, which my little legs could not step up, so I crawled! This step led up to the kitchen, where just about everything was going on. The blacklead range was huge, much bigger than ours; it had two sway poles instead of one. Auntie cooked breakfast on the range, using home-cured bacon and mushrooms picked straight from the field in the autumn. I remember one time when Auntie gathered some mushrooms the night before and left them peeled on a plate overnight. The next morning, though, all she had was a plate of holey mushrooms as one had had a grub in it, and the grub had happily munched away on the other mushrooms overnight! There were no mushrooms for breakfast that morning!

My Auntie and Uncle used to cure their own bacon, and during the Second World War my Auntie had to appear at the Dore and Bredwardine Magistrates' Court for selling bacon on the black market. She was let off with a caution, though, as the police could not prove their case. The bacon was always very fat and most of the rasher would melt in the pan, so that all you ended up with was a small piece of very crispy fat bacon. On the other hand, you might be offered some home-cured ham, which was taken from the back leg of the pig and was out of this world taste-wise. However, on this visit I was not to be tempted; I was still not eating, being very ill with presumed whooping cough.

On each side of the fireplace there were two armchairs, not the type you have today, but the wooden variety with two wooden arms. They were very comfy, especially with a cushion on. You toasted your home-made bread on a long-handled toasting fork in front of the fire, scraped a meagre amount of butter onto it, and then resumed your seat to enjoy your toast. I absolutely adored home-made butter, but even toast and butter could not tempt me now. I was getting thinner and thinner.

Also in this vast kitchen was a water pump which pumped up water from the well. Seemingly this was not fit to drink, because the same system as at home was utilised, and water for drinking was fetched in two buckets from a well across the field. This well was tucked into the hillside and had a small wooden lid on it. You only fetched enough water for drinking purposes. It's a wonder we all survived, because the farm's sheep also drank from the well! The pump in the kitchen at The Kellyn was for washing purposes only. We never took a bath while we were there, but I suppose the family did so, as a tin bath hung on the wall identical to the one at Yew Tree Cottage.

Uncle and Auntie at The Kellyn also had an outside toilet. This one was even further away from the house. An expedition to their toilet meant going out through the back door, across the grass yard, and down a sort of path to the end where the toilet was situated. This meant an even longer and colder journey on winter nights. Every bed, however, had a 'goesunder' – a chamber pot in case of emergencies in the night. Like ours, Uncle and Auntie's toilet was a one-seater and was placed over an outflow from the cattle yard. Of course, there was a wall separating the two. Toilet paper at Auntie's toilet was 4" squares of old *Hereford Times*.

Off the kitchen was another dark cold room, called the dairy, where Auntie separated the cream and made butter and cheese. She would spend many hours separating the milk in a separator. The cream would be sold at market. The process of separating the milk was very technical. Milk would be placed in the separator in a large metal bowl at the top, and a handle was turned, operating a complicated set of pipes and fittings. After the handle had been turned furiously, making a funny whirring noise, the cream would come out of one pipe into a bucket and a watery residue would come out of the other pipe. This residue was fed to the pigs with meal which had been ground from corn. Auntie would also make butter from the spare cream. This involved putting cream into the churn, which is a barrel-like appliance with a handle. The barrel was rotated by turning the handle until the cream turned into a solid mass, which was the butter. Most churns in those days were referred to as 'up and over' churns, and the process could take hours to complete. It was usually better to make butter on cooler days, as in the hot weather the cream would not turn to butter.

Once the cream had turned into butter, a thud could be heard as it turned in the churn. There was great excitement once this happened as the butter had 'come', and there was not much more churning to be done. The only thing now was to add more cold water and continue to churn for a short while to wash the butter. Then it was time to take the butter from the churn, add salt to taste, and then form it into a pat. The patting was done using a pair of Scotch hands, two pieces of wood with a pattern on and a handle on each, much like table-tennis bats. The salt was never measured, but Auntie would make remarks like 'Butter's a bit salty this week' or 'Didn't put enough salt in this week'. Butter was weighed into half-pound lumps and patted into oblong pieces, and had ribbed effects along the sides. It was then packed into greaseproof paper and put in the cool, waiting to go to market in Hereford on Wednesday. The dairy was a lovely cool place, wonderful on hot sultry days.

Also in the dairy, Auntie made her cheese. Now I never did see this being done, but there was a huge array of cheese presses, handles and levers in this room. Cheese-making involves the introduction of rennet, which is a by-product from a cow's stomach. This revolting stuff was also used to make junket, which I shall mention later in my story.

The Kellyn farm wasn't far from the Black Mountains and as a treat one day Auntie said, 'Shall we go whimberry picking?' All agreed and we set out, except Uncle, armed with our baskets. Now, whimberries go by several different names, but whatever you call them they are very, very tiny. It takes an awful lot of whimberries to make a tart – and a lot of sugar, as they are very sour. These little berries grow low down on bushes hugging the mountainside. I can still picture the scene of all of us setting off down the mountainside with our baskets, having accomplished our goal of getting enough whimberries for our pie. As some of you will know, mountainsides get very slippery with dry grass in the summer, and the rabbits nibble off the grass too, making it very short and slippery. This was, I fear, the cause of the next disaster, as my mother, complete with her basket of whimberries, slipped and fell, upsetting all of her haul! She immediately burst into tears, but everyone simply set about picking up the whimberries. How many we lost, and how many rabbit droppings we acquired, I will never know! But back at the farm the pie was duly made and enjoyed by all.

Uncle and Auntie had a very hard life at The Kellyn, bringing up a few calves, chickens, ducks, etc. Uncle also had a small garden, but it was a thankless task, as most of the soil on The Kellyn ground was near to the rock, making it impossible to grow anything much. He did, however, grow lovely strawberries, the lovely Alpine type, similar to the wild ones.

When I was a little older and stayed once again at The Kellyn, I was usually asked to let the geese out of the shed in the yard. Now geese terrified me, and I would stand behind the door and let them out. Ganders are extremely ferocious. There was always a tremendous flapping of wings and squawking. They would run and half-fly all the way up the yard, past the pool, and then take to a semi-flight down into the valley below where the Dulas Brook flowed. At night, they all strolled dutifully back to the shed in the yard. Fortunately, the ducks were a different matter. They were much more sedate and spent most of the day swimming in the pool in the yard.

Uncle and Auntie did not own a car as neither of them could drive. If they travelled, they usually went on foot, by bicycle or on the bus to Hereford on Morgan's buses. Wednesday was market day in Hereford, and Morgan's put on several buses into Hereford. Everyone knew everyone on that bus, and later in my life I would go to stay with Auntie and Uncle and travel into town on that bus. The bus was usually full with a menagerie of animals, people and luggage, baskets etc., etc. There were boxes of chicks, dead rabbits, hens in cages – you name it and it would be on Morgan's bus from Longtown to Hereford on a Wednesday. The passengers would climb aboard with their assorted foods for market. The driver would know most of his passengers, and many a time he would have to wait for Mrs So-and-so, as she was just changing into her market shoes from her wellies or taking off her pinny.

Sometimes, someone would arrive on the bus with their slippers on! If you'd changed from wellingtons, you would leave the wellies in the bottom of the hedge – upside down, so they'd be dry on your return from town. We always had the welly changing saga, as we had to cross a field from The Kellyn to the bus. Where the bus stopped, there was a stone stile which had been there for generations.

All around The Kellyn there were footpaths to and from the other farms and to the road to catch the bus. Usually, the stiles were made from a large stone block, similar to a gravestone. It was one of these which we used to climb over to get to the road. They were very stockproof, as little lambs could not climb through them.

The nearest shops to The Kellyn were either at Ewyas Harold, Longtown or Pontrilas. This meant either walking or going on your bike. Bread was usually baked at home, but, if not, the baker would call twice a week. His name was Mr Allard and he was from Peterchurch. He delivered for miles around the foothills of the Black Mountains. The butcher also called a couple of times a week and took your order during the week for delivery on the Saturday. There was no telephone at The Kellyn, but Prossers at the farm next door, called Old Court, had a telephone. Legend had it that there was an underground tunnel between Old Court and The Kellyn. I always imagined a door opening in the house to reveal a black passageway. It never happened! The only public telephone box was on Lower Maescoed Common, and the exchange was called Longtown Castle; what a lovely exchange name!

The landscape in and around The Kellyn was very beautiful and is indeed still beautiful and unspoilt. In later years, after I had recovered, my cousins and I would go down to the bottom field by the River Dulas. The water was crystal clear, and as both my cousins could swim they often donned their costumes and bathed in the lovely deep pools which the river made. It was a romantic and exciting place, with dark trees hanging over and huge boulders to clamber over. I would sit on the boulders and watch my cousins having a wonderful time in the river and dip my feet in the crystal-clear water. Other than that, I would take jam jars and turn over stones to find the little fishes which lived underneath, and transport them home to The Kellyn.

On our journey to the river we would pass a field which had clumps of golden wild daffodils in the spring months. Later in life, I would gather armfuls of these lovely flowers, clutching them to me as we walked home. Also by the River Dulas was a mill house, which was occupied by Mr and Mrs Moses. Mrs Moses had only one eye and terrified me when she stared at me with her one good eye.

Watercress grew well at The Kellyn, and I developed a liking for the peppery hot taste, which is most enjoyable in sandwiches or in salads. In those days it was said that it was not advisable to eat watercress when there was no 'R' in the month as it had large, bossy flower heads, so watercress was not eaten between May and August. In the months with an 'R' in them, the watercress was OK to eat and was young and tender. There was an area just to the side of the well we used for water which had an open trough. This was fenced off from the sheep, but we shared the water in which the watercress grew. Again, it is a wonder we didn't catch something from the sheep. Today's watercress is grown in controlled situations with pure water running through its roots. However, when I was on my holiday, I felt so poorly that even watercress sandwiches made from home-made bread, butter, watercress and salt didn't tempt me.

Dad joined us at the end of our holiday, and soon it was time to go home to our cottage at How Caple. Time had moved on and we were into August.

Chapter 6

Diagnosis and the County Hospital

We travelled home from The Kellyn to How Caple, first on Morgan's bus to Hereford Bus Station, and then to Yew Tree Cottage on the Midland Red bus.

On seeing us arrive home, Mrs Gordon hurried across the road. It was only couple of hundred yards from her house to ours. She held a note in her hand which she read out to Mum and Dad, as her writing was illegible. The message was that Dr Malkin from Fownhope wanted them to get in touch with him regarding my illness. He had obviously been giving my condition much thought while we had been away, such was his concern for me.

Mrs Gordon offered the use of her telephone. Dad did not like telephones at all and, right up until his death in 1991, he avoided using them if he could. Mum telephoned Dr Malkin, who advised that the results of the X-rays taken at the hospital a fortnight before were not good. He asked Mum if she and Dad could take me into the County Hospital in Hereford for further X-rays and to see the specialist in lung complaints, Dr Phillip, as soon as possible. Once again Mum and I set off on the dear old Midland Red bus.

The bus station in Hereford is very near to the County Hospital. The plans for the County Hospital had been developed in the early 1930s. It was a three-storey-block hospital to provide accommodation for 115 patients, including advanced cases of tuberculosis. Both the City Council and the Hereford Trades Council expressed their concern at having a hospital in the centre of Hereford which could treat tuberculosis patients. However, the County Council's public health committee, which was responsible for the planning of the new hospital, insisted that the best advice possible had been obtained, both medically and architecturally, and the risks were minimal. The hospital site was duly approved and Queen Mary, on her visit to Hereford on 29 July 1937, laid the foundation stone. The hospital, which would be known as the County Hospital, Hereford, was built at a cost of £68,836 by Messrs Bowers and Co.

There was a ward called Nightingale Ward (which was to treat tuberculosis and midwifery isolation patients). This ward was spread over two floors and was named after Florence Nightingale, who did so much to enhance the training and status of nurses. There was also a children's ward called Christopher Robin, after A A Milne's character in the *Winnie the Pooh* stories.

When Mum and I arrived at the County Hospital, we were immediately sent to the X-ray department for another X-ray to be taken. This X-ray was to prove to be much quicker than the X-ray which had been taken a fortnight previously. It was a Saturday morning and, after the X-ray had been taken, we were ushered into Dr Phillip's room. I was oblivious to what he was saying as I was only five years old, albeit coming up to six; but what he did say to Mum was that I had miliary tuberculosis, that it was serious and that there was no cure. Whatever must my poor mum have felt at the time? What was the future to hold for her little girl, her only child? She must have felt extremely frightened and upset, and I suppose in deep shock, as any mother would be. She told me that her reaction was one of disbelief that her only daughter was so ill. When she gathered her thoughts and wits together, she told me that she replied to his statement that I was so seriously ill by shouting at him,

'No, no! You're all ruddy wrong! How dare you say this about my child?' She rarely swore, but who could blame her?

When things calmed down a little, Dr Phillip said not to take me about too much. What did that mean? Was it because I was so ill, or was it because I was infectious? I learned much later that tuberculosis is very infectious. He went on to say that later on, perhaps in a couple of weeks, they would get me a bed in hospital for care. My mum enquired about the prognosis and whether I would get over it. Obviously she had not taken in his original statement that there was no cure. She also asked what miliary tuberculosis was, and she was told that it comes from the word *miliarus*. It wasn't patches on the lungs, it was spots, millions of them, and *there was no cure*. Dr Phillip made no mention of how they proposed to treat my illness. Was I going to hospital to die? Who knew the answer to this question?

In the early part of the twentieth century the spread of tuberculosis was becoming increasingly recognised. When associated with loss of weight, it was referred to as 'galloping consumption'. Many cases involved children under the age of five. From 1908, Public Health Acts placed the responsibility on county councils for the notification of cases of tuberculosis and the provision of facilities to treat children.

We both returned to the security of Yew Tree Cottage on the bus. Mum was silent for most of the journey, although I suspect she would have been trying to act normally. How did she tell my Dad? I was the apple of his eye, yet his 'Rowy' (his pet name for me) was going to die! My dad was a sweet, loveable man; he had a very simple approach to life. How would he cope with this most terrible news?

Human nature is peculiar in that as soon as people knew that I had tuberculosis it was as if they had a leper in their midst. Tuberculosis was thought to be a disease of dirty people, although this was very untrue. My mum had asked

Dr Phillip at the hospital how I had contracted this disease, and he said that it was impossible to confirm how, but it could be milk, as this was a time when milk was not tested for tuberculin. Was that third of a pint of milk, which I loved each day at school, to blame for my illness, or the local delivery of milk to the door daily? There were so many questions which remained unanswered.

I continued to do all the things that children do. I played with my dollies and other toys and I can't remember feeling particularly ill, just very tired.

I had contracted whooping cough in spring 1947 and had only been at school for two terms. I hadn't yet learned to read and write. I was off school the term between Easter and the summer holidays, and we were now in August 1947. The County Hospital administrator sent a letter saying that I should now be admitted to the County Hospital, and I went into hospital on 8 August 1947. Dear Mrs Gordon took Mum and me in her car to the County Hospital where I was left – all alone! They both then returned to How Caple, Mum having left her only daughter in the care of doctors and nurses, not knowing the outcome; but it looked very gloomy indeed. My mum, dad and I had never been parted!

I had a room of my own in this newish hospital. It was clinical and felt cold, even though it was centrally heated. There were other rooms on this floor similar to mine containing other patients whom I would never meet. If I left my room and stood in the corridor, I could look out over the bus station and watch the buses. The first lane was used by 'Red and White', the second and third by Midland Red, the fourth by Morgan's and the fifth by another bus company. This was my only occupation, bus-watching! That, or just lying in bed. On the far side of the bus station was the Ritz Cinema... so many bricks in that wall, hundreds of them! This was indeed a distressing day both for me and, of course, Mum and Dad. Why had they left me in this place? I remember crying copiously, sobbing my heart out, wanting Mum and Dad. I was so very, very lonely and upset. This loneliness was to increase further over the next few weeks. I was so isolated from the other patients that I even had my own toilet with a label on it which said 'Rosemary Only' – was I a leper? Was I really unclean? Little did I know it, but worse was to come in my long struggle against ill health.

In those days, of course, mums and dads were not allowed to stay. How very different it is now! It was so cruel to separate a child from its parents. The hospital protocol was such that nursing staff took care of children, and parents were only allowed to visit on Wednesday, Saturday and Sunday afternoons, and only then for an hour.

The décor of the ward was clinical; everything was white! The staff were starchy and stiff, with set uniforms and little white hats. They showed very little love. Now, don't get me wrong, they were never cruel to me, but they just nursed. I never got dressed and wore only my nightie and dressing gown and was extremely frightened. I was so frightened, in fact, that I didn't ask for the toilet and once soiled the bed. I was so ashamed, even at five years old, and am still ashamed to this day. I have never told anyone until now and can see that solid mass in the bed even today.

I had my sixth birthday in that place, but there is no memory of it, absolutely no memory at all. Was I too ill? Did I have a visit from my mum or dad or my beloved gran? Did I have a cake or presents? I simply can't remember. There are those questions in my mind again.

As I have said, the staff were not unkind, but there was no love. I was just left in a starchy white bed, alone in this little room for hours on end, with only the occasional visit from a nurse bearing a kidney-shaped bowl with the barrel-shaped syringe in it. These injections of penicillin were given to try to cure the tuberculosis, but little hope was placed on it working. It was literally a shot in the dark. The only consolation of having had all these injections is that I now have no fear of needles. Apparently I never cried when having the injections, I just took it all in my stride. If you remember, my mum had been told that there was no cure, *no cure*. It was like clutching at straws in the wind, so the doctors said.

I had regular visits from a nurse bearing a bowl of water, flannel, soap and towel who then gave me a bed bath. This was done each morning. One vivid memory of this dreadful place was that of taking a normal bath. This was not a regular performance, but having been in bed so much I had developed bedsores, or boils, on my legs and body, and I was indeed a sorry sight. The nurse would run a bath and put something in the water which was yellow in colour; I suspect now that it was iodine. When I was placed in the bath from my wheelchair, I screamed out loudly due to the pain which was caused. I still bear the scars of the bedsores on my legs to this day, and I was chastised for crying!

A couple of weeks after I had been admitted, the hospital was quarantined because of a poliomyelitis outbreak. No visitors were allowed in at all, not even parents or grandparents. How I missed my mum and dad! I also longed to see my gran, she was a lovely 'cuddly' gran. I make no mention of my granddad, as I never saw him.

I gather that Mum made frequent visits to the hospital hoping to see me, but on getting to the offices on the second floor marked 'Sister' she would be denied entry to the ward, and on enquiring of my health she would be told I was 'comfortable and going on well', but she was still not allowed to see me. How dreadful for her – to be that close but still not be able to see me! What a terrible thing, to be denied the only reassurance she could gain from seeing her daughter. I suspect that the staff just didn't think of my mum's anguish at not being able to see me. She was terribly worried and went home crying to Dad that they might not see me alive again.

It was on one of these desperate days that my mum approached the sisters' office and asked to see Dr Phillip for an update on my condition. She was told that he was away and she took this information to be correct. She walked back down to the front door on the ground floor to be met by the porter, whom she had grown to know and talk to over the previous weeks. He could see that she was upset and asked her what was wrong. She blurted out that she wanted to see Dr Phillip but that he was away. The porter, surprisingly, told her that indeed he was not away but had, in fact, just left the building. Was Dr Phillip hiding from her or afraid to tell the truth? Were the hospital staff protecting him from a distraught and angry mother?

On another occasion, after one of her fruitless visits to the hospital, she was, first of all, pleased to see our local priest, Reverend Wynne Thomas, standing on her doorstop. She had not seen me for some considerable time, nearly a month in fact, so you can imagine that she was absolutely furious when he said, 'I've been to see Rosemary and you will be pleased to know that she is relatively well.'

Her anger spilled over and she let fly at this poor unfortunate man, saying, 'Why have you been able to see Rosemary when I haven't been able to see her for nearly a month? I'm the child's mother!'

His reply was that as he was a man of the cloth and was allowed access to places where others were not. Her retort was that because he was a man of the cloth, as he put it, that did not give him any more rights than any other person. His clothes could still carry germs into the hospital, and she asked him how often he washed his suit! Not often, I suspect; he apparently left with a flea in his ear – man of the cloth or not.

Spurred on by the Reverend's visit to see me in hospital, my mum, on her next visit, insisted on seeing Dr Phillip. He informed her that I was stable at the present time, receiving penicillin, but when I became very ill, I would die. In fact, he said, that would be in less than two months' time. He told her that there was very little hope.

On hearing these words, my mum expressed her concern that neither my dad nor her were able to visit me, and Dr Phillip said he would try to do something about that fact.

Chapter 7

Nieuport House

One Wednesday, 1 October 1947, a few days after my mum's visit to see Dr Phillip, a letter arrived at Yew Tree Cottage, quite out of the blue.

The letter informed them I was being moved from the County Hospital to Nieuport House, a sanatorium for tuberculosis patients, near Kington in North Herefordshire. I was getting further and further away from my beloved parents and my little home. In that letter, Dr Phillip told Mum and Dad that I appeared to be getting better and my health was improving. This letter gave Mum and Dad a little more hope than they had had previously.

I was taken by ambulance to Nieuport House. By this time I was well used to being bundled about, but wondered where I was going. Dr Phillip had asked Mum to organise some clothes for me to use at Nieuport House, and all of these clothes had to be marked with my name. There's that stigma again – infectious disease! What the letter did not say, though, was when I was going to be moved, but it must have been at about the same time as the letter was sent to my mum and dad. Mum and Dad decided they would visit me at the Nieuport Sanatorium on the Sunday after they received the letter. Little did they know that I had already been moved to my new hellhole, Nieuport House. Had I been sent to Nieuport House to die?

Nieuport House is situated in a small village called Almeley and the earliest document which mentions Almeley is the Domesday Book of 1086. The first house built on site was built in Norman times and was called Newport House, but over time it became Nieuport House. One of the most distinguished owners of the property was Sir John Oldcastle, who in all probability was born there in 1360.

During the reign of Charles I, Almeley was bought by Francis Pember, one of the richest merchants of the time. From then on, Almeley was owned by families of merchants and industrialists, many of whom made their fortune in the North but found recreation in the peace of rural Herefordshire. In 1774 the owners of Almeley rebuilt Nieuport House and its external appearance remains more or less unchanged to this day.

In 1917 the Nieuport Estate came into the possession of Herefordshire County Council. The land was split up into fifty-acre units and leased out to veterans of the First World War. In the 1920s, Nieuport House was converted into a sanatorium and £9,500 was spent converting the house and stables into units for patients. There were 62 beds – 18 for men, 16 for women and 28 for children.

A subcommittee of up to twelve members was appointed to supervise the administration of the sanatorium and the grounds. On 29 January 1923, Nieuport Sanatorium was opened, most patients having lung tuberculosis, which was judged curable with the use of drugs and fresh air.

There were some children there who were ill and malnourished and had been admitted to the sanatorium for observation, not because they had been diagnosed with tuberculosis themselves, but because they had been in contact with relatives or friends who had been diagnosed with tuberculosis, and their malnourishment was a possible symptom of the disease.

From its opening, Nieuport Sanatorium provided outdoor schooling and employed a teacher. There was a cinema, a sanatorium magazine and a snooker room. Part of the stables was used to house the sanatorium's one-ton Morris ambulance. In the 1930s, Dr Ainslie had brought his mobile X-ray unit to the sanatorium at a cost of £5, but towards to end of the 1930s a permanent X-ray department was installed on-site. Nursing tuberculosis was dangerous, and over the years three nurses died after becoming infected.

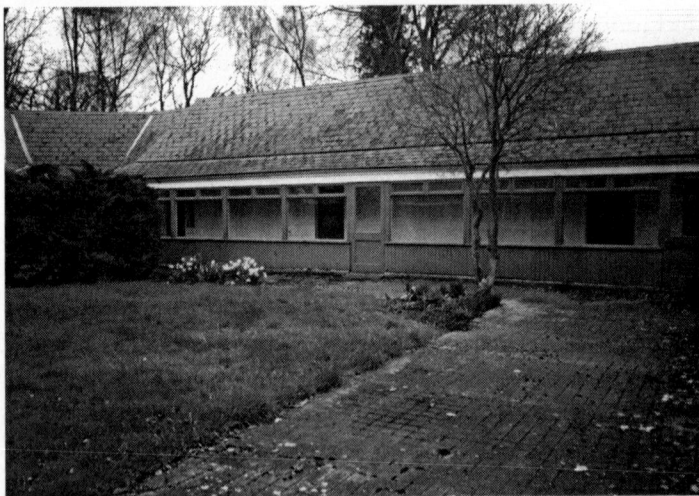

Nieuport House in 1999 (now with closed-in veranda; in 1947 it was open)

Nieuport House was presumably where I had been deposited to die, although thankfully, as I was still so young, I didn't realise it.

Mum and Dad had arranged a visit to see me at Nieuport House on Sunday, 5 October 1947; however, things were to take a dramatic turn on Thursday, 2 October.

Mrs Gordon had been into town in her car and had called in at the local post office. The two Misses Bundy ran the post office and they told Mrs Gordon that they had just received a telegram for Mr and Mrs Webb (Mum and Dad). They asked if Mrs Gordon would deliver it. Mrs Gordon agreed and, as Mum was working at The Cross that day, she took it straight to Mum. The telegram read:

CAN GET ROSEMARY ADMITTED TO BRISTOL CHILDREN'S HOSPITAL TOMORROW FOR STREPTOMYCIN TREATMENT. STOP. STRONGLY ADVISE ACCEPT THE OPPORTUNITY. YOUR CONSENT RE-QUIRED. STOP. IF IN DOUBT, TELEPHONE ME AT HEREFORD 3029 BETWEEN 2 P.M. AND 5 P.M. SIGNED DR PHILLIP.

Mrs Gordon let Mum go home. She started to get lunch and waited for Dad to come home to discuss this new development. Dad returned from work at the Chapel Farm to find Mum crying into the potatoes over the stove. He thought instantly that his precious daughter had died. Dad asked what the matter was and, after Mum had explained, he said, 'Whatever are they thinking of? What are they [the medical team] going to do next?' The two of them talked over the contents of the telegram. They decided that I must go to Bristol. It was my only chance of life, and anything was better than nothing!

Mum went back to Mrs Gordon's to use the telephone, as they still had not got one. Dr Phillip's receptionist asked, 'Are you letting her go? It's her only chance, you know?'

Mum, who was a very strong-willed woman, said that she would only talk to Dr Phillip. She did speak to him, and gladly gave her consent to my move, to give me a stronger chance of survival. Dr Phillip advised that I would be moved from Nieuport House to Bristol the next day – Friday, 3 October. Mum said to him that she and Dad still wanted to see me, as they had not been allowed to see me for weeks. Dr Phillip said that if they could get to Nieuport House that day, they could see me. Mum advised him that they could, although she was a little surprised to hear that I was already at Nieuport House, They had received the letter telling them that I was going to be moved, but no one had told them that the move had already happened. Can you imagine not seeing your only child for weeks on end? It wouldn't happen now in the twenty-first century, but it happened then in the twentieth century! It was barbaric and cruel to have been denied access to your child for so long.

Dad hurried off to tell his boss, Mr Calvert at Chapel Farm, of the developments, and that he and Mum were off to see me at Nieuport House that very afternoon, as they had been told a car would meet them from the Hereford to Eardisley train to take them to Nieuport House.

Things would have to be carefully organised. We didn't have a car and the buses were very infrequent. So what happened? How did they get to see me? Well, my Mum, before her death in 2008, told me all of these things which she had rarely spoken of before.

It was Mrs Gordon who that day became a saint, she had a car and some precious petrol coupons (a legacy left over from the war), and she drove Mum and Dad to the train station at Hereford (about nine miles) where they caught the train to Eardisley, which is about three miles from Almeley. There had previously been a line between Eardisley and Almeley, but that had long since been discontinued, so they were met at Eardisley Station by the driver from Nieuport House, as arranged, who took them back to the sanatorium to see me. Mrs Gordon had reassured them that she would meet them at the train station to take them home again later that night, no matter what time it was, and that she was only a phone call away.

On their arrival at Nieuport House they were escorted into an office, where they met the doctor and staff in charge of my case. They were offered tea and were asked if they could sign the papers to allow my move to Bristol to receive the streptomycin treatment. Streptomycin was a new and untried wonder drug which was being given to the British people by the American government to trial. My mother always mentioned 'lease/lend' by the American government, but she said she didn't understand it fully, and never did understand the politics of it. Then, to their surprise, as this is what they had travelled all that way (thirty miles) at short notice for, they were asked if they would like to see me! Surely, that was such a silly question! They confirmed that they would see me and then sign all the papers.

I vaguely remember Mum and Dad coming to see me in my new hellhole. It is said that unpleasant things haunt you and that is very true. The conditions they found me in were very unpleasant. Had I really been put there to die? Mum has told me since then of the state in which they found me. I was in a deplorable state, I hadn't been washed for days, my poor little body was covered in bedsores, sores and boils, my hair hadn't been combed for days and it was matted and lacklustre. The doctor had come into my room with Mum and Dad and, once again, he asked if they would sign the papers. My dear dad, who was such a gentle man and never lost his temper, replied, 'She has to go somewhere, anywhere out of this dreadful place. She may as well die at home with comfort and dignity… We'll sign your papers!'

The ward at this dreadful sanatorium was in a block of converted stables which were all set round a quadrangle. The floor of the quadrangle was made of bricks set on their sides – like tiles. The converted stables housed the children with tuberculosis; boys in one part and girls in the other part. The adults were accommodated in the main house. I was only there a short while, so I never saw or visited the main house. The little rooms in the converted stable housed two or four beds. The rooms were a single room deep and only had one storey, except the doctors' house, which was two storeys high and set right in the middle of one of the sides of the quadrangle. Also in the quadrangle was the school house, the ambulance station, which housed the green private ambulance, and a dining room. There was also a mortuary in the main house. The door of my room looked out onto the quadrangle and was never closed. There was a glassless window at the side of the room. The fresh air was supposed to help with the treatment of TB. This glassless window looked out on what seemed to me to be some sort of wood or spinney.

As I have said before, I hate the wind and these trees were like evil fingers poking their way into my world through those glassless windows. I was literally terrified when I was there, just lying there with the sheets clutched up around my chin. I was terribly cold and couldn't understand why my parents, who I thought loved me dearly, had sent me there. I still shiver when I think of it – I was so terrified, and remember the room to this day. The room was sparsely furnished with just two iron beds; one was mine but the other was empty while I was there. There was a wardrobe, a dressing table and that dreadful little white enamel potty under the bed. The bed was so very uncomfortable; the mattress was made of horsehair and there were white sheets, a blanket and eiderdown. There was an en suite of sorts – a proper toilet and a washbasin, which was found in a little room off the bedroom.

When I arrived, I had no idea how long I would have to stay. Fortunately it was not long, just about a week, but the time I did spend there will haunt me for the rest of my life. The experience of being kept in that place cannot be described and, as I remember it now, it still sends shivers down my spine. Were the smells the smell of death? Imagine placing a child of six in conditions such as these. In today's society, social services would be summoned immediately, and the child taken into care if he or she were treated like that; but then the health authorities did it and got away with it!

I don't remember receiving any treatment here – or much attention, for that matter. A nurse did wash me occasionally, but not often. Mostly I was left alone in that room, with no enthusiasm from staff to stimulate me into having a will to live.

Mum recalls that after they got over the shock of finding me in such conditions on that fateful visit on that cold, early October day, with frost hanging on the trees, she took a comb from her bag and did my hair. It was so wonderful to have her loving hands on me again. She produced a ribbon and carefully placed it in my hair on the right-hand side. Tears are welling up in my eyes while I write this, I felt so wretched. She and Dad must have felt wretched too. I loved my mum and dad so much, but children are always closest to one parent or the other, and I was always so very close to my dad.

Was the Bristol Children's Hospital to be my salvation? They hoped so, but there were things to do before I left that place, like signing those papers they kept on about.

Out of the blue, the doctor in charge asked my mum and dad if one of them would like to accompany me to Bristol in the ambulance. There wouldn't be room for both of them. Arrangements were made, and Mum, who had been nominated to accompany me, arranged to meet the ambulance in Ross at the bus station at 9 a.m. She could catch a bus from How Caple to Ross, but it would mean an early start for both Mum and me. Mum said that come hell or high water she would be there to go with me.

Mum and Dad bade me farewell that night and left me to the mercies of the staff and that awful room.

They made their way back to How Caple that cold night. I wonder what they said to each other on the journey. It was a long journey: car to Eardisley, train to Hereford, and then a train to Fawley Station. Mrs Gordon had said she would pick them up to take them home, but this was not necessary as she had contacted Gran and Granddad Jones and told them of the fast-moving events of the day, and they were waiting at Fawley to take Mum and Dad back to Yew Tree Cottage. The conversation was probably very confused, but possibly a little optimistic at the events which were about to take place.

Friday, 3 October 1947 dawned frosty and cold again. The ambulance personnel were busying themselves around the old-fashioned bull-nosed green private Morris ambulance which had been seconded to the sanatorium. It was being filled with that precious petrol and oil ready for our journey to Bristol. It had a bell! The ambulance stood in the quadrangle just outside my little room. The ambulance man was dressed in a navy-blue uniform with a peaked cap and was very kind. That sight is the one I remember most vividly (and it is a very bright memory) of the time I was at Nieuport House – that and, of course, the white enamel potty!

At about 8 a.m., or earlier, we set off: the green ambulance, the ambulance driver, a nurse, me and that little white enamel potty – just in case! We headed towards Ross, where we picked up my Mum. On getting into the ambulance, she noted that the ribbon she had placed in my hair the previous afternoon was still in the same place. I had neither been washed, nor had clean clothes been put on me – a discovery totally alien to any loving mother. We went to Bristol via Gloucester, as the Severn Bridge had not then been built. It was a long, long journey down the good old A38.

I don't know how long it took to get to Bristol. I remember, though, seeing the view out across the Severn Estuary and the posh houses outside Bristol. I had to use that wretched little potty, but I suspect that the adults crossed their legs until they reached Bristol or a café somewhere. There were no services like those that today's travellers enjoy, and it would be another twenty years until the first motorway would be built.

Chapter 8

Bristol Hospital for Sick Children

Our sad little load must have reached Bristol Children's Hospital at about lunchtime, but this fact escaped me as, when you are a child, you have no concept of time, and as I was so ill it didn't matter to me what time it was.

The Bristol Hospital for Sick Children was perched high on a hill overlooking the busy and historic city of Bristol. The hospital originally had thirty beds, an emergency operating theatre and a casualty department, which had been installed only a few years before my arrival. The hill on which it is built is called St Michael's Hill and it is very, very steep. Buses and other traffic would often falter at its steepness as vehicles then did not have such sophisticated engines as they do today. The road is very narrow, and there are little flights of steps all the way down one side of the hill so that pedestrians can get up and down. The hospital was built of sandstone in an E shape, with large windows, three storeys high. There were other outbuildings adjoining it, containing departments such as X-ray and outpatients. Across to the left there was a huge bomb site, a remnant of WWII, with ghostly vacant-eyed buildings looking across to the hospital. There were craters littering the ground and wild plants springing up everywhere, mostly buddleia, as this usually thrives on poor, neglected sites. I don't know if the hospital still stands or not. I did read once that it was going to be demolished and a new children's hospital, with state-of-the-art facilities, was to be built elsewhere in Bristol, but I don't know if that actually happened.

We approached the hospital from the bottom of St Michael's Hill, its steepness making the old green ambulance groan. The ambulance parked on the street outside the main doors, facing uphill. All of our belongings were gathered up (except for that dreadful potty!) and we all processed into the hospital across a wide pavement and then up about ten steps onto a level platform-type area. There were then even more steps. These steps had a low stone wall on each side and behind these walls were shrubs.

The sad little procession headed into the hospital building. The ambulance man carried me, wrapped in a blanket, in his arms; the nurse followed behind us; and finally Mum brought up the rear, carrying my belongings. I remember that the nurse and ambulance man were chatting in hushed voices. One of the remarks made by the ambulance man has stuck with me all this time. He said, 'Such a pretty little thing, I wonder if she'll ever come out.' Even on hearing this I was not frightened, as to be anywhere other than Nieuport Sanatorium was a blessing.

I seemed to have been carted and bundled about for months. Was this my last resting place, good or bad?

Things here were to prove very different from the Herefordshire institutions. The hospital was, in fact, complete luxury. Even though Bristol Hospital had experienced severe bombing in WWII, the bombs had missed the main building, despite its very conspicuous position. Temporary repairs had been carried out so that its good work could continue. The main parts which had been affected were the extremities, the X-ray and outpatients departments. In 1947 a temporary outpatients department was built, but it was very cramped; most of the services were being provided out of huts, with several doctors sharing a room – one doctor in each corner of the room was the norm! In January 1947, internal alterations had been carried out to the hospital so that it could accommodate sixty children. Most of the doctors and nurses were in training as it was a training hospital.

The Medical Officer of Health for Bristol writes in his report dated 1947 the following: 'Deaths from Tuberculosis (all forms) in 1947 amounted to 241.'

Dr Campbell Faill, Senior Chest Physician, reporting on tuberculosis wrote that:

> Occasionally one gets gratifying results with injections of gold and sanatorium treatment, but at the best they are left with permanent damage to the lungs and nearly all show a tendency to sudden relapse. Possibly streptomycin may have some effect on this type of case and when larger supplies are available it certainly should be tried.

Our little procession trailed along the wide corridor with its stone floor and steps, which seemed to bend to the left until we reached Ward 5 which was to be my home for the foreseeable future.

Ward 5 was on the ground floor and the first ward on the left of the E-shaped building. There were six wards on three levels at the front of the hospital, all facing the heart and centre of the city of Bristol. These wards had a wonderful view. Ward 5 seemed like a huge ward after my solitary confinement at both the County Hospital and Nieuport Sanatorium. I was with other children and had none of the isolation previously endured. The ward had a fireplace with a fire halfway down on the left, and a bathroom and toilets at the corresponding point on the right. There were twelve beds, three on each side before the fire/bathrooms and toilets, and three on each side after the fire/bathrooms and toilets. The whole ward seemed so bright and cheerful.

The beds were still the old iron beds but they were so much more comfortable than those at the County Hospital and Nieuport Sanatorium. They had cast-iron headboards and footboards. At the far end of the ward, overlooking Bristol city itself, there were two very high glass doors with glass and brick from floor to ceiling each side of the doors. These doors led to another room, similar to the conservatories of today. This room was quite unique in that it had railings along the front, open to the elements (the railings were about three-feet high), a ceiling (which was the floor of the ward above) and a back wall. Once again the fresh air was supposed to help in the treatment of TB. The two remaining walls were made of glass and brick. This room housed another six beds, three on each side. I had been allocated the first bed on the right after coming through the doors. This is where I first met Michael Mallock, who was to become my friend. He was in the bed to my right. I also met a girl called Kathy in this ward.

The outside ward was obviously equipped with central heating as there were radiators on the back wall, i.e. the wall adjoining the main ward, or we would simply have frozen to death. I was soon installed in my bed with just a nightdress, bedjacket and dressing gown. We also wore bedsocks to keep our feet warm. The ambulance man and the nurse bade their farewells to me, but they allowed my mum to stay for a minute to have a private farewell while they waited in the office. I wonder if the ambulance man ever knew that I made it!

I snuggled down feeling safe, secure and, funnily enough, happy – a feeling I hadn't experienced for many weeks. I thought that it was a lovely place, totally different from Nieuport Sanatorium. Nothing could have been any worse than that place. The staff were lovely and friendly and I was made to feel very welcome. In those days, nurses wore different colours, with a little white starched hat with grips to hold them on. The sisters wore blue and also the matron. Both sisters and nurses wore a large blue belt with a large buckle. When out in the town, nurses wore lovely blue capes with red linings.

After leaving me in the care of the nursing staff, Mum went to have a word with the doctor in charge, a Dr Beryl Corner, and the sister on the Ward, Sister Valerie Hughes. There was also another sister, whom I grew to love, who was called Sister Owen. I will mention her later. I was formally admitted to Bristol Children's Hospital, bearing the number 1492 from Yew Tree Cottage, Hew Caple (not How Caple), on 3 October 1947.

Admission Details

No	Age	Name	Address	Admitted	Discharged	Contributory
1492	6	Webb, Rosemary	Yew Tree Cottage, Hew Caple, Hereford	3/10/1947		0.1

Apparently, Mum did not take to Dr Corner in the first instance as she accused my mum of neglecting me because I had all those bedsores, was unwashed and my hair was in a mess. This was like a red rag to a bull, and Mum swiftly put her right, telling her that I had not been in her care for weeks but instead had been at the County Hospital and Nieuport Sanatorium, and that it was their fault that I was in such a state, not hers!

The ambulance crew returned to Ross and deposited Mum at the bus station for her to return to Yew Tree Cottage. I wonder again what her feelings were on that journey, as she must have worried about whether her precious and only daughter would recover from this dreadful disease. I was now totally in the hands of medics, science and faith. It must have been a very lonely journey from Ross to How Caple on the bus, and an even lonelier walk that night from Cross-in-Hands to Yew Tree Cottage, along a narrow, dark country lane.

I settled in well and loved my new surroundings. Treatment started that very day with an injection of streptomycin in my bottom.

The other two beds in my section were occupied by a little girl called Kathy and a lad called Michael, whom I have mentioned before, and we three were soon friends. I didn't mind the fresh air, and to this day enjoy being out in the open with the rain on my face – not that it rained on our faces, you understand, but our feet could have got wet on many occasions! To avoid wet feet at night, the staff would come and check on us and put a big waterproof blanket on the bed; if I can recall correctly, I think it was red in colour. In the morning it would be covered in puddles of rain, and sometimes covered in snow! We would flick the rain and snow off the blanket, much to the annoyance of the staff, who would get an unexpected shower.

What did we do with our days, you ask? Each morning the staff would wake us, if we were not awake already, and give us a wash or sometimes take us to the bathroom for a wash; this was a real luxury for me, having had to endure the treatment I got at the County Hospital and the Nieuport Sanatorium. We would clean our teeth with tooth powder. The pink tooth powder was in a little tin and you had to mix a little water with it to make it into a paste.

Then would come a most awful procedure, which I remember with dread and hate. Along would come Sister bearing a kidney-shaped bowl with a red rubber tube in it. The whole lot, however, would be covered over with a cloth. I had to have this tube put down my throat and mucus would be brought up from my lungs. I hated this procedure so much and hate the thought of it today, but I put up with it and never complained. I doubt, however, that I would be quite so compliant if I had to have it done today!

Then we had breakfast, usually cereal and toast, although I can't remember what we were given to drink, probably milk.

Mum, Gran or Auntie Gladys used to send or bring us eggs for breakfast, and the nursing staff would boil one up on the ward. We usually shared whatever goodies appeared, and we all loved our boiled eggs and soldiers. We usually spent our days in bed watching the world go by. There were toys in the playroom and we would spend some of our time in there. In our ward there were two little twin girls who were very pretty and their father was extremely rich. One of the twins was called Carol, but I cannot remember the name of the other twin. Their father was very kind and would keep the ward well stocked with the latest additions to the toy world. There were little ride-on horses which, when they were pedalled, would move along. There were also ride-on roundabouts which seated two people and were great fun. Each child sat on a little seat by a handle and as you rotated the handle, you went round around, sometimes at a great rate of knots! We also spent time painting magic pictures and painting in pre-printed painting books. I loved painting and, in my later life, I have developed a love of watercolour painting.

Other than the toys sent in by the twins' father, we didn't have many toys, but I do remember having one of those bird whistle things into which you put water and, when you blew into it, it whistled like birdsong. There was also one of those birds which you placed with its beak over glass of water and it drank. However, to enjoy using these, someone had to go to the bathroom to fetch the water!

We were always allowed out of bed if we wanted to get up and were well enough to do so, except in the early afternoon when we all had to have a compulsory nap.

In those days there was no TV and there was no radio on the ward, so there was very little to entertain us. The nurses were very kind and chatted to us, played with us and read to us when they had time. There were a few books, but as I had only done the preliminaries for reading these were of little use to me. Michael, who was older than me, read a lot.

At one time during my stay some teachers were brought in to give us lessons in the late morning but, just as I was beginning to enjoy this learning, it suddenly stopped, and we never did find out the reason for this. Perhaps the prognosis for us TB children wasn't good and was judged to be a waste of time. Who knows?

The doctors usually did their rounds in the mornings and, as it was a teaching hospital, there were usually quite a few trainee doctors tagging along. Lunchtime was the highlight of the day. I can't remember much about what we ate, but minced beef and potatoes with vegetables was one of my favourites. It was plain, basic and wholesome food.

At regular intervals I was approached by the nurse or sister carrying the kidney-shaped bowl and syringe containing the streptomycin. The nurses were so skilled at their job, they just dabbed some cold substance on my bottom and injected. I never felt a thing. I didn't mind the injections, but the morning ritual involving the rubber tubing caused me much distress. I had the injections four times a day, if I recall correctly. My skin sometimes resembled a pincushion and new areas had to be found to inject! I had to have a blood test about once a week. I remember once that the nurse could not find a place in my arm to take any blood from and she had to take it from my ankle. That was painful! Even to this day, my veins are difficult to get blood from. I wonder if that is because of all the treatment and injections I had all those years ago?

We took tea, or supper, which would usually be sandwiches or cream crackers with butter on them, at about 6 p.m. My Auntie Gladys would send me a parcel with home-made butter in it and the nurses would make me up cream cracker and butter sandwiches. For pudding we usually had blancmange or junket. This slimy pudding will stick in my memory for ever. I hated it, but the staff insisted that we 'eat it all up, as it would do us good'. It is made out of rennet, a by-product from a cow's stomach, and milk and flavouring, but it was horrible and slimy. Our drinks mostly consisted of milk or flavoured milk. At night we were given a hot drink and perhaps a biscuit if there were any. Remember, this was during the post-war years and there wasn't much of anything around.

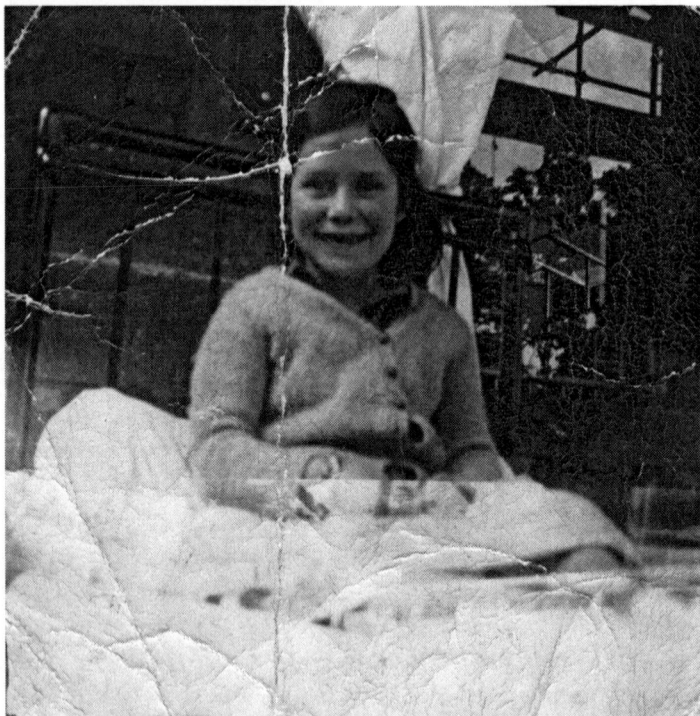

A few days after my admittance in October 1947

From our vantage point high over Bristol at the top of St Michael's Hill, we could see all or at least most of the city. It was a wonderful sight, especially at night, because we could sit and watch the lights gradually being switched on, all different colours, a very magical sight. On one such night as we were watching, a pall of smoke and flames crept into the sky – Bristol Hippodrome was on fire!

In front of the ward was a small green lawn with a weeping willow in the centre and, in the spring, up would come crocuses of every shade and colour. Now, when I see crocus in spring, I am reminded of that ward in Bristol Hospital. Smells do the same – remind you of when you first smelt them.

I had been brought to Bristol Hospital for Sick Children to hopefully be cured of miliary tuberculosis. The American government had given the British government eighteen beds' worth of treatment of streptomycin, a new wonder drug – untried and untested, but full of hope for curing tuberculosis. No one knew if it would work, but our hospitals in England were trialling it. There were six beds in London, six in Birmingham and six in Bristol. If it had not been a gift, the treatment would have been very expensive, apparently about £2,000. The National Health Service was being talked about but it would be another two years before it was formed.

A child had died in Bristol and I had been given his/her place. Dr Corner emphasised to Mum that if that child had not died I certainly would have, but that they were going to do their best to get me better. It would take a very long time, but hopefully the treatment would be successful. The child who died in Bristol died that I might live! I never knew whether it was a boy or girl, but I was given a chance thanks to that unknown child.

On my admission, my mum was asked by Dr Corner if they would allow a post-mortem to be done if I died. What a decision to make! But she made it and signed the papers, hoping that they would not be used.

I have one awful memory of my time on that ward and that is of having to have a lumbar puncture done. I do not know if this was because they were worried I had meningitis, or whether it was because of my illness, but this was an extremely painful procedure and in those days there were not the painkilling drugs of today. All I can remember is extreme pain.

I was placed in new bed near the toilet entrance facing towards the entrance door and told to lie on my side and to keep *very* still. The staff even held me down. I was extremely frightened. A very large needle was then placed into the centre of my back and I believe something was drawn off. I never did know the technicalities of it, but it was awful. I did as I was told and it was soon over, thank goodness. A bad memory day!

As Bristol was a teaching hospital, about once month we were all taken, complete with beds, next door to an annexe of the hospital. We all then lay or sat in bed and had doctors explain to their students what was wrong with us all. The students would then examine us, prod and push us and do various things to advance their training as doctors. I did not like this procedure very much and didn't look forward to these teaching events. Indeed, one evening – these exercises usually took place in an evening – I burst into tears and got very upset and was taken back to Ward 5. I remember my fellow patients arrived back some time later!

Once, there was great excitement on the ward. We were to have a visitor – Uncle Mac (Derek McCulloch) from the BBC. He was a children's radio presenter. I vaguely remember him, a tall thin man, who gave us all a book entitled *Uncle Mac's Own Story Book*. I have it to this day, and my granddaughter loves me to read it to her.

In those post-war years, there wasn't much fruit about. We rarely had it on our menu for lunch or tea. Now, as luck would have it, my maternal Gran's brother, Charlie, and his wife, Ellen, lived in Old King Street in the centre of Bristol, in Broadmead. Both Gran Jones and Auntie were called Ellen.

They owned a greengrocery shop in Old King Street, which was within easy, albeit laborious, walking distance of the hospital. Owning a greengrocery business meant that fruit was no problem to them. Their little shop had missed the bombing by inches. The factory behind the shop had been bombed, and the towering factory with its blackened charred windows was a very eerie sight on wet drab days. The shop was like an Aladdin's cave once you had climbed the three large steps to get into it. It had a dusty wooden floor, worn thin in places from the continual human traffic, and was stocked with everything from turnips to Tizer. Charlie and Ellen's living quarters were through the shop at the back, with stairs going up through the middle passageway. They had a sitting room and a dining room, and right out the back there was a sort of conservatory. It was a huge, glassed area, stocked to the ceiling with gigantic foreign ferns growing in large wooden containers. They had two bedrooms upstairs and, luxury of luxuries, a bathroom and a flush toilet!

Uncle Charlie and Auntie Ellen were a lovely old couple; at least they seemed old to me, but they were, in fact, only one generation above my mum and dad.

Uncle kept most of his stock upstairs, above the shop. In those days, bananas were a rare sight. If any appeared, which they would in Bristol as this was the first port the fruit came into after the Second World War, Uncle would remark that he was 'just going out to the banana plantation to pick a bunch or two'. In fact, he kept the green bananas, which had come off the boat at the port, on the stairs, which is where he ripened them.

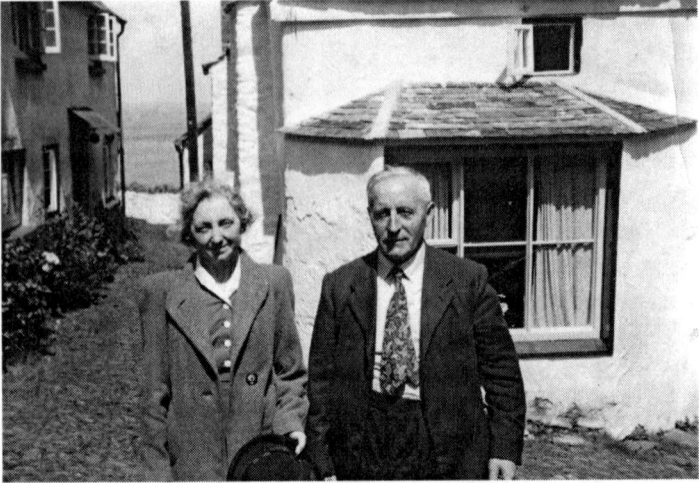

Auntie Ellen and Uncle Charlie

Meanwhile, back home at How Caple, Mum would go to Hereford, our local market and county town, on the bus on a Wednesday and look in shop windows at children's basic post-war clothing. She would shed a silent tear and not risk purchasing anything, as the clothes might not fit me or, worst of all, might perhaps be wasted.

Visiting arrangements at this new (to me) hospital were much more liberal, but being so far away, Mum, Dad and Gran could not come as often as they would have liked as it was very costly. Even though Gran and Granddad had a car, Granddad was afraid to drive in a city as big as Bristol. Either Mum and Dad or Gran and Mum would visit about once a fortnight, as it was a strict two visitors to a bed policy, bearing goodies such as puzzles, comics, picture books, etc. Each patient had a table which could be pulled up over the bed, much the same as today's bed tables. We would do our puzzles and painting on those. Parcels would also arrive from Mum and Dad or Gran, or Auntie Gladys at The

Kellyn. There were also food parcels with biscuits, cream crackers, butter (yes, *butter*), eggs (however did they stay in one piece?), ham and chickens ready to roast. The staff would roast or cook anything that came in and we children had a lovely time. Anything was exciting, and things to eat were especially good to a little girl of six who was, by this stage, feeling much better and getting her appetite back!

Whoever visited from home would have a long and complicated journey, firstly getting on their bikes to go to Upton Bishop to catch the bus to Gloucester. They left their bikes at Wallin's of Upton Bishop, who were the local bakers and shopkeepers and friends of our family. Mum knew them well and, in due course, I would become friends with their daughter, Sue, real name Elizabeth. At Gloucester they would sprint across town to catch the train to Bristol (Temple Meads).

At Temple Meads, which was a beautiful building, they would once again sprint across town to Uncle Charlie and Auntie Ellen's in Old King Street, and after saying a quick hello they would then walk up that awfully steep St Michael's Hill to the hospital. They would, after visiting me, return to Old King Street, and sometimes stay there for the night if they were too tired to travel or had missed the last train to Gloucester.

One very vivid memory of my stay in Bristol was when my Great-Auntie Ellen, who was a very tiny lady, visited me. A murmur would go around our little group out in our balcony ward that 'Rosemary's Auntie' was coming across the lawn. In those days there wasn't the security that there is these days, and she would, when she had time and things to bring to me, come struggling up that hill to visit me. I can still see her standing there with a brown paper bag (no plastic in those days) in her hand, peeping through the vertical railings, her tiny face and head nearly coming in through the gap. She really was a tiny lady. Her bag usually contained goodies such as fruit and sometimes sweets. She then proceeded to push the goodies through the railings. This ritual was, however, destined to come to an end, as a child was kidnapped and killed in another part of the hospital, so a wire mesh was constructed from floor to ceiling for security.

The night the child – or baby, I think it was – was kidnapped, we 'outside residents' watched all the commotion outside on the lawns and around the buildings. I vividly remember the police with torches hunting round us. It was very exciting for us children, but not so exciting for the staff and authorities. The workmen arrived soon afterwards to barricade us in, thus curtailing Auntie Ellen's clandestine visits! After this, Auntie had to come the more conventional way through the main doors and then from the main ward into our ward. Everyone enjoyed Auntie's visits, as we all shared whatever came. She would bring those precious bananas, which tasted so much better than the ones you get these days. We were all extremely happy in that ward.

When the centre of Bristol was redeveloped in the 1950s, after the bombing, Uncle Charlie and Auntie Ellen had to move out of their little shop. They retired and were rehoused on the outskirts of Bristol, and Uncle Charlie was able to develop his love of gardening. He only had a pocket handkerchief-size garden out back at Old King Street, with those bombed-out factories looking down on it. He did, though, have an allotment out at Coalpit Heath where he grew vegetables, but it was a bit of a struggle getting out there because he did not have a car and had to go there and back on his bicycle. He would, however, take a bag with him and bring back whatever vegetables (even though it was like bringing 'coals to Newcastle'!) and flowers he could. He loved to grow flowers mostly, especially roses. Auntie Ellen was allergic to all types of primulas, i.e. polyanthus, primroses, etc., so he never grew those. Mum would take Auntie, when they were at Old King Street, a bunch of flowers from the garden at Yew Tree Cottage, making sure though not to include any primulas!

After the redevelopment of Bristol, the only thing left in Old King Street was the chapel. Which denomination it was, I cannot remember, but there was a horse and rider statue outside, with the rider missing his stirrups. It's funny the things you remember! I think the John Lewis department store building (ship-shaped in design) stands on top of what was Auntie Ellen and Uncle Charlie's greengrocers!

While I was at Bristol Children's Hospital in 1948, there was great news. Quads had been born at Southmead Hospital and 'my' doctor, Beryl Corner, was both a paediatrician at Bristol Children's Hospital and the inspirational doctor responsible for the newborn babies at Southmead Hospital. These were the first set of quads to be born and survive in the West. Their names were Bridget, Frances, Elizabeth and Jennifer Good – the Good Quads! This was before IVF.

The nurses and sisters in that hospital were so very, very friendly, and were especially trained to deal with children. We had a matron, mostly dressed in dark blue or black, then various sisters, various nurses and then the auxiliary staff. All were recognisable by their uniforms. They all wore an apron, stiff starched collars and, of course, a little starched hat, as mentioned before. When they were out in the town they wore a navy blue cape. These nurses looked so smart. However, I never encountered a male nurse at Bristol; maybe there just weren't any.

We were all X-rayed at least once a week. The X-ray department was across the road in the portable huts and a building which had escaped the bombing. This was a weekly treat. There were tropical fish over there, which we all loved watching. The nurse would load me into a wheelchair and we'd set off, turning left at the doors of the ward, into the corridor, which was very wide and stony cold. We passed other wards on the way and at the last corridor, which was very straight, the nurse would get up speed and we'd tear down the corridor like maniacs until we reached the end.

At the end there was a ramp and stairs down into the street. By now we were descending St Michael's Hill! We crossed the street, passed the fort and went down into more corridors and turned left into the X-ray department. We didn't usually wait about. I remember having to stand in front of the machine, cuddle it and hold my breath! Once the X-ray had been taken, we would do the return journey, still tearing like maniacs along the hospital corridors. I was so much happier here than at Hereford County Hospital or the Nieuport Sanatorium.

The outpatients department was also housed over the road by the X-ray department where there were dozens of fish tanks. I loved to watch them; they are very therapeutic.

The Bristol Hospital was my home for ten months until August 1948, when I made another move, this time to a home by the sea – Burnham-on-Sea, in fact. I was to move to Jan Smuts Convalescent Home at Burnham-on-Sea in Somerset (it was a part of the Bristol Children's Hospital). I went there with a nurse and, this time, we went by car, not ambulance. Mum was, once again, asked for permission for my move, which was gladly given as it was one more step towards my recovery.

The course of treatment of streptomycin had finished, the blood tests were needed less often, the X-rays were improving and generally my health was much better. It was felt now that I needed to convalesce.

Chapter 9

Jan Smuts Convalescent Home, Burnham-on-Sea, Somerset

Once again I was off to a new home, this time to hopefully find a complete cure from that dreadful disease, tuberculosis. At this home I would make new friends and reacquaint myself with some old ones. The day I left Bristol Children's Hospital, I left on foot, walking side by side with the nurse who would accompany me to the convalescent home. I clutched my belongings tightly, but when we reached the front door where, all those months ago, I had been carried in, not expected to live, I dropped a pot of cream which I had been given to treat the eczema which had developed. I don't know whether it was nerves or what that made me drop the pot, but I was very upset. The nurse, however, cleaned up the glass and cream, which had spread all over the place, and gently reassured me that it did not matter and I would get another pot of cream.

The journey did not take long. Burnham-on-Sea is on the Somerset coast, just west of Bristol. We arrived safely and, once again, I soon settled into my new home. The Jan Smuts House was built of brick and set in Berrow Road in lovely gardens, about a mile from the sea. In 1945 the Trustees of the South African Aid to Children Fund presented the house and £2,000 (to spend on adaptations and repairs to it) to Bristol Children's Hospital. I do not know anything about Jan Smuts other than that he was a South African politician of that time, and the house was named after him. The secretary to the fund, Mrs Keightley-

Smith, was living in Burnham-on-Sea at the time, and naturally took a great interest in its development. It had opened in 1946 with twenty-three beds.

The house was built in a pre-war design with bay windows facing out onto the gardens. There was a level piece about 3 to 4 yards wide along the front, which led down to a large piece of lawn about the size of a tennis court with flower beds. In summer, the toys would be brought out to the front piece of grass for us to play with. The back looked out onto the dunes and the golf course, which we walked across to get to the sea. There was a shrubbery at the back and a longish private drive.

My new home was lovely and, even better, it had a garden, which I loved! The rooms were quite large and there were four or so beds in each room. It turned out that later on I would be joined by my good friend from Bristol, Michael. Our room overlooked the garden through one of the large bay windows. The regime at Jan Smuts was much more leisurely; we didn't have to get up so early and could have long lie-ins if we wanted. All our meals were taken in the large dining room at the back of the house. After lunch we still had to have a rest, which had to be taken by lying on a mat. There was no excuse, the rest was compulsory. It seemed like we'd lie there for hours, but in fact it was always only about an hour. There was no talking allowed at this time, just rest! Very often we would all fall asleep, so I suppose the rest objective had been achieved. If you weren't tired, however, it was very boring as there was no music to listen to and the mats placed on the hard wooden floors were terribly uncomfortable.

It was here on 17 September 1948 that I was to celebrate my seventh birthday. Mum and Dad visited me and brought me some clothes for my dolly, Susie. We had a cake for our tea, although things were still scarce in those post-war days. Susie had been acquired for me by a lady called

Mrs Williams who ran a little café in Broad Street in Ross-on-Wye. I loved Susie very much. She had a lovely porcelain face and eyes which closed when she was laid down. Sadly, Susie came to a tragic end years later when Dad accidentally dragged her out of the car and her beautiful face smashed (as she had somehow become attached to his mac belt), and Mum, misguidedly, threw her out – much to my disgust when I asked her later in life what had happened to Susie!

A few days after my birthday, one of the nurses wrote a card for me to send home to Mum and Dad. It was a Mabel Lucy Attwell cartoon card with a little girl taking a bath on it, dated 19 September 1948. The very neat writing on the back of the card reads:

Dear Mummy and Daddy,

Uncle is going to send me a parcel. I had a lovely birthday and we all had tea together on a big table.
I am hoping to see you again. I still love my dolly and take her to bed every night. I am feeling very well.

Love, Rosemary xxxxxxx

At Jan Smuts House I was allowed to wear day clothes, i.e. a blouse, skirt and cardigan and shoes and socks. We were able to use the house and gardens freely, and enjoyed just playing and running around the gardens every day. The autumn was closing in, but I was so happy to be feeling better and be out in the air. We were, however, never allowed out of the grounds. One day I caused a terrible scare. I cannot remember whether it was autumn, winter or spring but, on this occasion, I forgot all sense of time and started to chat to some children over the fence at the bottom of the garden. Little did I realise that a search party had been organised and they were all out looking for me. I casually strolled back to the house, having missed my tea, and received a very stern telling-off!

As at Bristol, we were all able to wash daily. The bathroom was at the bottom of the stairs and we all lined up, boys on one side and girls on the other, all clutching our towels and wash things. There was a huge white cast-iron bath in the middle of the bathroom with enormous taps. We were washed in turns, and I never did find out if they changed the water for each of us! As well as the bath, there were two flush toilets in the bathroom; each had a long chain with a cast-iron cistern fixed high up on the wall. The shorter people among us had to jump up to catch the wooden handle as it swung to be able to flush the toilet.

There was none of the fresh-air treatment that I had experienced at Nieuport House and Bristol. The only fresh air we got was when we were out playing, and we had the choice of whether to go out or not. All in all, it was a lovely place for children. There was a huge playroom with a plentiful supply of toys for all ages.

I became very attached to Sister Hughes at Bristol and Sister Owen at Burnham-on-Sea. I was very lonely at both of these places, despite the company that I had, and I missed my mum dreadfully, so I clung to these two as if they were my surrogate mums. In later years, Mum told me that the fact that I clung to them so much when she left me after her visits upset her very much. I suppose in my mind Mum had abandoned me, and I looked for a mother figure to give me love and comfort when I needed it.

By this time I had become very institutionalised. I had grown used to being with other children and I was very independent, as I am today.

The time I had spent in Hereford County Hospital, Nieuport House and Bristol Children's Hospital had led me to become bed bound, so I had to do exercises with my feet, which had become a funny shape due to my being in bed for so long, and in fact they never regained a nice shape.

Sister Owen wrote a letter to Mum and Dad regarding this problem:

Jan Smuts Convalescent Home
Burnham-on-Sea
29.9.48

Dear Mr and Mrs Webb,

Rosemary is going ahead well – Dr Mason saw her yesterday and was very pleased with her.

She seems awfully happy and was so pleased with the dolly's clothes. Nurse has helped her with a letter which has probably arrived by now.*

She is having exercises each morning for her feet which seem to help a lot. She gets up about 10.30–11 and has a rest after dinner. She is longing to go for a walk by the sea, but it's a little bumpy over the fields, so I have said that perhaps next week, we might go.

I shall look forward to seeing you on Saturday week.

Yours sincerely
D E Owen (Sister in Charge)

In a letter dated 22 October 1948, Sister Owen mentions our trip to Bristol for blood tests and X-rays. She also mentions some photos which had been taken and which she would send to Mum and Dad, and the fact that some shoes they had sent did not fit. It must have been difficult for Mum to buy shoes for someone who she only saw about once a fortnight at the most, and then only for short periods at visiting time.

The letter reads:

Jan Smuts Convalescent Home
Burnham-on-Sea

---

* I do not have this letter. Mum carefully kept all of the letters written by the staff during my stay, but some have obviously been lost over time.

22.10.48

Dear Mr and Mrs Webb,

Rosemary is going on well, they were pleased with her at Bristol on Monday. She thoroughly enjoyed her trip and coming back we had tea and cakes at a very nice restaurant and she was thrilled as were Kay* and Daphne.

I've got some very nice photos – which I am getting printed and will send on as soon as I can.

Rosie says thank you for her lovely parcel. She is thrilled with the clothes – the shoes unfortunately don't fit, but everything else does, very well.

The ham was lovely, thank you for sending it. We had a lovely supper and Rosemary has had several sandwiches which she enjoyed.

We still haven't been to the sea yet. The weather is so unsettled and showery.

Yours sincerely and love from Rose,
D E Owen

In another of those letters, Sister Owen asked permission of my mum and dad to have my hair cut, and requested a reply by return. I suspect that the mail must have been quite efficient, as Sister seemed confident that a reply would come before the hairdresser called.

> Jan Smuts Convalescent Home
> Burnham-on-Sea
> 26 October 1948

Dear Mr and Mrs Webb,

Rosemary is still going ahead well and is very happy. She likes to have your postcards, and sends her love to you both. It will be nice to see you when you come next time.

May I have Rosemary's hair cut a little shorter? It is so long and straggly, I think it would do it good – could you

---

* Kay is in fact my friend Kathy from Bristol.

possibly let me have a postcard by return as I would like to have the hairdresser this week.

Yours sincerely
D E Owen

A few weeks later a letter is written to Mum and Dad on my behalf. In the letter there is talk of toy horses which you sit on, and which move along when you pedal. These horses were similar to the ones at Bristol and were probably made by the manufacturer Triang. They had probably come from the twins' father, as the twins were also at the home at the same time as I was.

Another letter sent on my behalf reads as follows:

Jan Smuts House
Burnham-on-Sea
13.11.48

Dear Mummy and Daddy,

David and Cathy had a parcel with me today and we had breakfast in the playroom as the dining room is being painted, the playroom has just been painted and it's ever so nice.

I went for a walk with Nurse White and I saw some nanny goats.

We have three horses and you have to press the pedals and it goes along. We have got a nice big dolls house which we play with in the garden.

The doctor was so pleased with me, the painters are still here, they are all now painting the dining room.

Lots of love,
Rosemary xxxxx

On the reverse of the letter Sister Owen writes:

Dear Mr and Mrs Webb,

Nurse has written a letter from Rosemary so I hope you

don't mind my going on the other side.

　　She is still very well, and very thrilled with her parcels. She hasn't had the skirt on yet but is wearing it this afternoon, so will let you know how it looks, also the socks.

Yours sincerely
D E Owen
PS I hope you had a good journey home last time.

The next is a letter written, as if from me, by a nurse:

Jan Smuts Home
Burnham-on-Sea

Dear Mummy and Daddy,

Thank you very much for the lovely parcel. I gave everyone a sweet and am going to eat the rest myself. I am wearing my skirt which doesn't get dirty because I wear my pretty pinny. I like the magic painting books because you only have to use water. The playroom is being painted so we are in the dining room. Goodbye Mummy and Daddy.

　　Give my love to Lance, Percy and Irene and Maureen [cousins and godmother's daughter].

It must have been in one of those letters which went backwards and forwards between Yew Tree Cottage and Burnham-on-Sea that Mum must have asked if I could go home for Christmas. The reply from Sister Owen is set out in the following letter:

Jan Smuts Home
Burnham-on-Sea
Dec. 1948

Dear Mr and Mrs Webb,

I am enclosing the photos of Rosemary. I hope you like them. She is marvellously well and I have taken her down to the sea, at last, which she loved!

I have asked about Christmas but Dr Mason is a little dubious but I suggested that she might go home anyhow for a fortnight over Christmas and then come back but so far have not had a definite answer, but I am hoping it will be all right.

I am in rather a hurry so please excuse more.

Yours sincerely
D E Owen

The photos referred to above are on page 108.

It appears that the request for me to go home, at least temporarily, over Christmas was, despite high hopes, denied. The convalescent home was, however, a lovely place, and we all enjoyed Christmas. This was the second Christmas I was to spend away from my home at Yew Tree Cottage.

Burnham-on-Sea is a lovely little seaside town, and very often parties of several children and a nurse or two would be seen in the area out walking. Sometimes, though, we would catch a bus into town. It was a small town with only a couple of main streets and the accompanying shops. I recall that just before Christmas 1948 we all went into town to do some Christmas shopping. We travelled in by double-decker bus. After our shopping trip we were all waiting very patiently at the bus stop to catch the bus back to the home when it started snowing. We all gazed skywards, looking at the magical blobs of snow. This is one of the vivid memories I have of my time at Burnham-on-Sea.

In the letter below, the nurse writes on my behalf that I had done some weaving. I remember the weaving, but we also did 'French' knitting. You can buy manufactured French knitting kits these days, but back then we made do with an old cotton reel with four little nails hammered into it (as it would have been a wooden cotton reel) at regular intervals, a needle and some wool.

Jan Smuts House
Burnham-on-Sea

Dear Mummy and Daddy,

Just a few lines to let you know that I am feeling fine and hope to be home soon. During the last week the nurses have taught me how to weave and I have made you a nice mat in all different colours. Guess who came down last Tuesday, Michael Mallock, Ann and Gillian. It's ever so nice having Michael down here. He sleeps in my room by the window. When we go to bed at night we lie in bed and talk of what we did in the hospital.

Michael's Mummy has just come down to see him.

I can do the jigsaw ever so quickly now, I think it is ever so nice. Well Mummy I will close now as it's nearly time for tea.

All my love to you both,
Rosemary xxxx [signed by me]

The New Year of 1949 arrived and life continued as it had, with Sister Owen writing letters to Mum and Dad either on my behalf or simply about me:

Jan Smuts House
Burnham-on-Sea
14.1.49

Dear Mr and Mrs Webb,

I seem to have a few moments with nothing to do! So thought I would write a few necessary letters.

Rosemary is going on very well and doing all she should. I think she has written to you. It is Kay's birthday next Wednesday so we shall be having a 'do'. I feel I must thank you again for the chicken you sent us at Christmas and for all the eggs you gave sent at various times; I do appreciate it so much.

Rosemary's auntie sent her some butter a few days ago, if you write, say 'Thank You'. They all love it on cream cracker biscuits.

Monica was pleased with her postcard, she was thrilled to pieces to have something by post. Thank you for thinking of her.

Yours sincerely,
D E Owen (Sister)

So this time it was Kay's turn for a party. They were a frequent event at the home.

Sister Owen's letter referred to my having written to Mum and Dad. It appears, however, that this was not done until the next day:

Jan Smuts House
Burnham-on-Sea
15.1.49

Dear Mummy and Daddy,

This is just a little note to thank you very much for my lovely parcel. I was very pleased with it, we all ate the chocolates on the sand dunes this morning while we were out for a walk.

The other day I pulled out one of my bottom teeth and put it underneath my pillow. The next morning I found a sixpence under there which the fairies had left me.

I hope you will like the weaving I'm sending you, perhaps you could make yourself a purse out of it. I am in the middle of making some more so when I have finished it, I will send it to you or bring it home with me when I come.

This afternoon Michael Mallock's Mummy and Daddy came to see him so he was very pleased.

This week I had a big parcel of butter from Auntie Gladys so we have it on biscuits for our tea.

I must close now as it is tea time and I have to be washed.

With lots of love,
Rosie [This one I signed myself, albeit a bit wobbly]

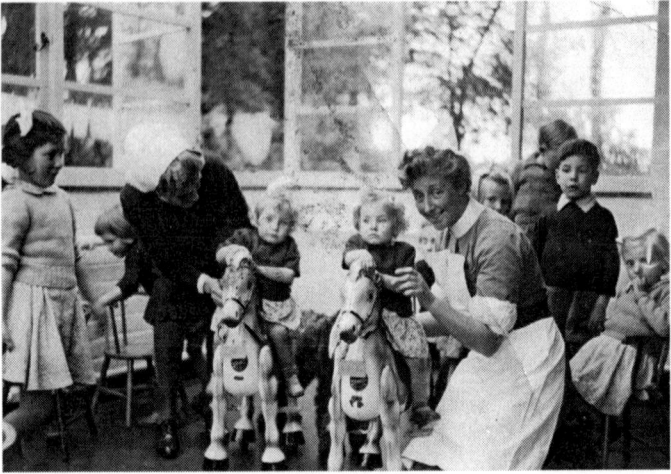

Left to right: Author, Cathy (Kay), Sister Owen, Twins (one of whom was called Carol), unknown sister or nurse, unknown, unknown, David, unknown (but there is a Monica referred to in the letters and this may be her)

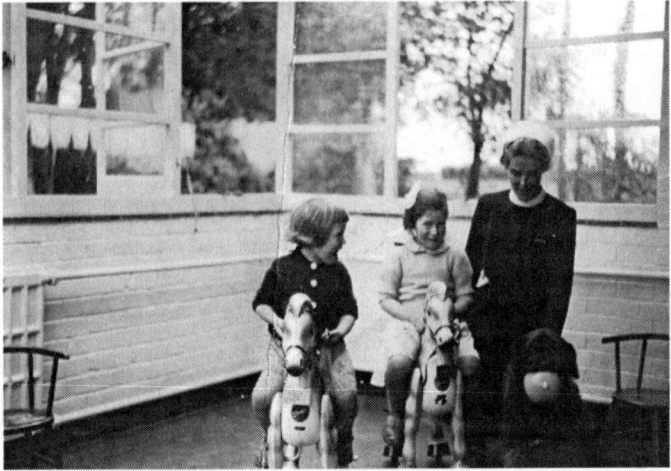

Left to right: Cathy (Kay), author, Sister Owen, and a dog

Life went on, with each day more or less the same as the one before it. We had visits from the doctors at Bristol and went for shopping trips and walks with the staff. We spent hours just playing with toys, generously supplied by the twins' father, either out in the garden or inside the play-room. We also made frequent trips up to Bristol for X-rays, and usually called at lovely tea rooms on the way back. It was a leisurely existence. We had lovely meals and the staff continued to be so kind.

In the spring of 1949 we had a sort of fête or 'Open Day' event. We were all out in the lovely gardens and were spoilt rotten that day. The twins' father had just bought some more toys and we were all trying these out. He had also bought us some pink and white nougat, which we all loved, as sweets were still on ration.

Also at this time we would walk across the dunes and golf course to the beach and the sea. I absolutely loved these walks, and felt the sea to be so powerful and fascinating to watch. At Burnham-on-Sea there is a very interesting lighthouse, but not a conventional sort of lighthouse. It was built on the beach, was made of wood and had eight legs suspending it over the sea. I suspect that it was rebuilt often, as the sea could be very rough. Interestingly enough, there were two lighthouses. One was inland and disused and had been turned into a house, and then this strange eight-legged one. The one which had become a house was, by then, part of a large housing estate – so it wasn't much good to shipping!

Once, during one of our walks across the dunes to go to the sea, I came upon a small bird's nest with eggs in it, in a gorse bush. I was extremely excited and wanted to show it to everyone, but on our next walk several days later it had gone. My disappointment was evident and I was very upset. It is obvious to me now that a predator had been at work and had destroyed the nest and those lovely blue eggs.

On one occasion at the home I was taken very poorly, so poorly that I did not want to leave my bed. The doctor was sent for and I was confined to bed, which I hated. I suspect I had flu or some other childhood illness. The doctor had come from Burnham, as it was a long way for one to come from Bristol. I wasn't allowed outside at all during this time and longed to be with my friends.

Mum, Dad and Gran would visit as often as they could, but this meant travelling for hours at a time on a bus or a train, or both. Sometimes, as they had when I was in Bristol, they would spend the night with Auntie and Uncle at Old King Street in Bristol. The bus from Bristol to Burnham was a very slow way to travel because, as it was a local bus, it would call at every village along the way.

The following letter recorded my illness:

Jan Smuts House
Burnham-on-Sea

Dear Mr and Mrs Webb,

Many thanks for your letter and the parcel of butter that Rose had. She was very pleased with it all.

I do hope that you will be able to come on Saturday, we have hardly had any fog around here, and now it is sunny.

Rosemary is very well, at least she had a little sore throat for about 3 days but it seems to be clearing, several of the children have coughs which is a nuisance but not to be wondered at I suppose, with all our funny weather.

Hoping to see you on Saturday.

Yours sincerely,
D E Owen

Another letter recording my life at Jan Smuts reads as follows:

Jan Smuts Convalescent Home
Burnham-on-Sea
Wednesday

Dear Mr and Mrs Webb,

Rose had her parcel today and was very pleased with it, especially the painting book which she was thrilled with, she should do very well at school I think – she loves doing things and learning things. She enjoyed the [can't read the writing] too.

Isn't the weather cold – fortunately the sun has been shining but the wind is bitter.

Yours sincerely
D E Owen

Chapter 10

Going Home

An undated letter, which I presume was written sometime in late May or early June of 1949, arrived at Yew Tree Cottage. The letter read as follows:

> Jan Smuts Convalescent Home
> Burnham-on-Sea
>
> Dear Mr and Mrs Webb,
>
> Rosemary has gone to Bristol, she went up yesterday with Matron, I think she will be there a few days before coming home, her cough has almost gone, but Dr Mason wants it quite clear before she comes to you. Sister Hughes will write to you as soon as she knows the day.
>
> I can guess how excited you must be – Ann Tand has just gone home and Gillian will be the next. Kay as soon as their house is ready.
>
> The weather is wonderful too – absolutely ideal for children.
>
> We all miss Rosemary very much I'm afraid, but we shall look forward to seeing you if you do come to Burnham.
>
> I tried to put in all Rosemary's clothes – we haven't sent her blue sandals as they are rather trodden down at the back, and I think there will be a few extra socks to send on.
>
> All good wishes
> Yours sincerely,
> D E Owen

I remember being told I was going home. I was nearly eight years old. I had been in and out of hospitals of sorts for twenty-two months. Everyone seemed excited, and I joined in with the excitement that I was going home – whatever those words meant!

The reason that I was sent to Bristol was so that, after they had done some final blood tests, they could officially discharge me. I had travelled to Bristol in the hospital car and was, once again, given a bed in Ward 5. This time I was on the inside of the ward and the bed I was given was halfway up on the left, by the fireplace. I was more or less left to my own devices, playing with toys or chatting to the other children.

The blood tests, unfortunately, showed worrying signs, and my discharge was put on hold. I vividly remember standing by my bed trying desperately not to show my disappointment, but I was crying, with my worldly goods all packed up. As it transpired, though, further blood tests, taken a few days later, showed that everything was OK. Apparently, Mum was very worried that the TB was back.

Those couple of weeks prior to my discharge home were, as I recall, a bit boring. Once again I was paraded in front of trainee doctors and the like so that they could see for themselves what a miracle streptomycin was.

The final letter sent by Sister Hughes, dated 10 June 1949, informed Mum and Dad that I could, at last, go home.

Bristol Royal Hospital for Sick Children
St Michael's Hill
Bristol
Telephone 20138
10 June 1949

Dear Mrs Webb,

Many thanks for your letter. I have been waiting to hear from Dr Corner when Rosemary could go home. She has just been in to say Rosemary can go home on Monday next, June 13th, or any time after that at your convenience.

Rosemary is very excited at the prospect and is looking very well.

All news when we see you. No need to let me know when you are coming, I know how difficult these things are to arrange for you.

Yours sincerely,
Valerie Hughes

It was, in fact, Mum who took that final journey on 13 June 1949. She arrived at the hospital with my clothes and waited while a nurse helped me get dressed. She had brought a pinafore plaid dress and a jumper; these were a bit hot for June, but I suppose that she had thought it was better to be safe than sorry, and had not wanted me to catch a cold!

Someone took a photo of Sister Hughes and me outside the hospital. I do not know who the other patients are in the photo as, this time, I was only on a fleeting visit to Bristol! You can, however, clearly see the railings which Auntie Ellen used to peep and feed goodies through, and the wire mesh attached after that dreadful murder.

It was a strange feeling. I was leaving the hospital with my mum, but she was, by now, almost a stranger to me. She had come through those double doors to collect me, but told me afterwards that when she saw me carried in through those doors all those months ago she thought that the only way I would leave would be in a coffin, to be buried in the local churchyard at How Caple. It was so emotional for her. She told me later that she was crying when she came into the ward and, little did she know it, so was I.

We said our farewells to the staff on Ward 5 and made our way, once again, to those front steps of Bristol Hospital for Sick Children, where my life had been saved by the sheer devotion of the staff and the new wonder drug, streptomycin.

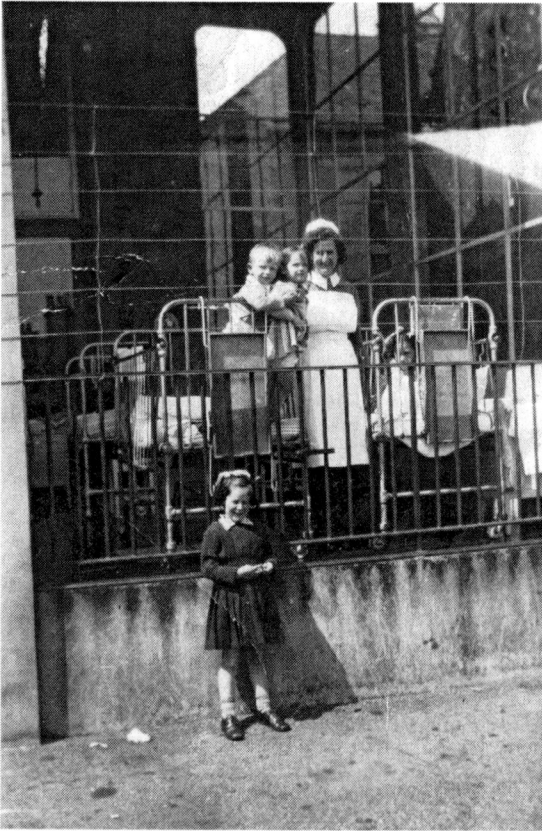

Going home – Ward 5, Bristol Royal Hospital for Sick Children,
13 June 1949 with Sister Valerie Hughes and 3 unknown children

The hospital car, which was waiting, took us to Temple
Meads Station. We went by train to Gloucester and then
changed to another train for Ross-on-Wye. At Ross Station
Mr Calvert (Dad's employer) was waiting in his posh car.
He drove us to Yew Tree Cottage, which was about six
miles away. We arrived at Yew Tree Cottage where Dad was
waiting – with the kettle on, I suspect. Mum and I walked

into the living room of that little cottage with me clutching my belongings. It was *so* small, the rooms were tiny, and it was all alien to me.

I was very frightened. Everyone had built me up to be excited, but the balloon had burst. To me this place was dreadful. I still remember standing there, not knowing what to do and feeling that I wanted to go back to Bristol or Burnham. I had been away from my little home for twenty-two months – nearly two years. Life had moved on for everyone. Where did I fit in? A considerable amount of adjusting would have to be done for all three of us, and 13 June 1949 was the start of that adjustment.

Chapter 11

Taking it Easy, School and Aftercare

So here I was, now living with two virtual strangers. I had to learn to live with them and to love them again. Sister Hughes and Sister Owen had been my family for the best part of the last two years of my short life, but Mum and Dad couldn't help that. They had saved my life by agreeing for me to go to Bristol on 3 October 1947. I had seen little of my dad over that time. He was such a lovely, gentle man who was loved by everyone who knew him. He would tell clean country jokes and always had his audience spellbound. It was, at times, difficult for the three of us to live together again. It wasn't difficult, though, to learn to love Dad again and I soon became his inseparable companion. Things were more difficult for me and Mum, however. I suppose that, in my mind, my mum had deserted me, as she was the one who had left me in those dreadful places – though, of course, this was not the case. It wasn't her fault.

During the summer of 1949, Mum and Dad discussed whether or not they could afford to buy a car. Dad knew of one which was for sale for £100. Dad had always been very careful with his money and had saved more than enough in his Post Office account. So the sum of £100 (a year's pay for some people in those days) was withdrawn from the account, and Dad proudly drove the little Ford 8 Series Y (black), Registration No. AWX 238, back home to Yew Tree Cottage. It had to be garaged at Mrs Gordon's, across the road, as there were two huge yew tree stumps up the drive to the cottage which could not be negotiated by car. These stumps would have to be removed before the car could come home. Dad had never taken a driving test; he was one of the few who had licences before the driving test was introduced in the 1930s.

I had been advised by the doctors that I could not go to school, and that I must rest and take it easy for several months before the thought of going to school could even be entertained.

Dad would drive his new car to various other farms in and around How Caple to do little jobs on Saturdays. These jobs included hedge glatting,* fruit picking, gardening and the like, and I always went with him. I usually sat in the car waiting for him or sometimes went in the house, depending on where he was working that day. My dad was not an educated man and liked simple occupations. He did not like working indoors and definitely would not have liked an office job. Mrs Gordon liked Dad to do the garden at The Cross, and when he went I would usually go with him and go into the house and chat to Miss Foster, Mrs Gordon's companion. She would let me help with the cooking. This was often a long process, as she was very particular and would have to have everything properly laid out before we even started cooking.

Mum still had her cleaning job with Mrs Gordon, and I accompanied her on a Tuesday and Friday morning. I can remember the posh smell of the polish and the smell of the proper coffee, which was still taken at about 10.30 a.m. The house had lovely big rooms with parquet flooring and I was allowed in all of them. The lounge was the room where the previously much-written-about telephone lived.

---

* Repairing gaps in hedges.

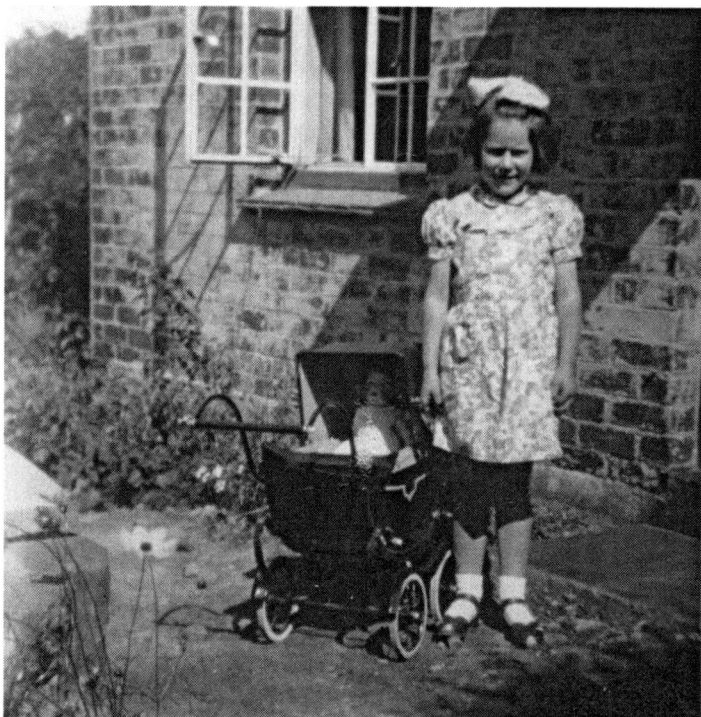

A picture of health
This was a 'formal' professional photograph taken, I think, on the
same day Dad had his photo taken with his 'Champion's Cup'
In the pram is 'Susie'

The Cross was very big and was built on the side of the hill at How Caple. At the front of the house there was a veranda built with stone slabs which had stone tubs and ornaments on it. There were lovely scented plants which crept out through the stones. It was a truly enchanting area. From the veranda, some wide stone steps led down to another part of the garden which was huge. It was like *The Secret Garden*! On the veranda grew summer honeysuckle, jasmine and all sorts of fragrant shrubs and plants. On hot summer mornings I would help Mrs Gordon do the flowers for the house, and that is one of the smells I wrote of earlier which will live with me for ever. She would do the flowers in a separate room off the veranda called the Garden Room. This room housed all the vases and materials needed to do flower arrangements.

One of the lawns at The Cross had Mrs Gordon's initials carved into flower beds. These beds contained lovely little pink and white cluster roses, which these days are called patio roses. Mrs Gordon's Christian name initials were 'J', 'L' and 'E'.

A little later, Mrs Gordon moved to a smaller residence at the bottom of How Caple called The Cottage. Ours was a cottage, but not like that cottage! Here Mrs Gordon had both a telephone and a television, yes, *television*, a nine-inch black-and-white set. In the mornings, for about an hour or so, there was a 'test' programme on. It was always the same, every morning, week after week. Mrs Gordon would sit me down in the lounge to watch it. I can nearly remember what it was all about. There was a large sailing ship or galleon, with a youngish man and a monkey. The story revolved around the young man's adventures on the galleon. I absolutely loved this treat and I never misbehaved, but just sat glued to the small screen. Mrs Gordon was incredibly good to both Mum and Dad throughout my illness and after – as, indeed, she was good to me.

Even with my Mum and Dad's company and some well-meaning neighbours, I was very, very bored and longed to go to school, as up until then I had only had two terms of schooling. I couldn't go, however, as I was at risk in case I picked up an infection which would set me back. At times, Yew Tree Cottage seemed like prison to me, and I missed my friends from Burnham very much.

The only highlight of the day, or so it seemed to me, was when Mr George Francis and his boys, Kenny and Bobby, came by in the evening with their half-dozen or so cows and calves. In those days, small farmers could not feed their cows in the summer months as the small fields had to be put up for haymaking. There was therefore nowhere for the cows to graze, only a small bare patch where they were penned with water during the day. Come the evening, the stock would be let out from their patch and they would graze the long acre – that is, the sides of the roads. Their long acre extended from Churchfields, which was their smallholding in Yatton, to Cross-in-Hands (where our little lane met the big B-road). The grass on the roadsides would become extremely short, especially at the Pump Corner, where our water came from. Mr Francis and his trusty band would accompany the animals, making sure that they did not get in anybody's garden or get involved with a car. The latter eventuality was less likely as we didn't often see cars.

With the Francis family, there was often a dear old gentleman called Jim Guest. He lodged with the Francis family. Jim Guest and his companions would dress more or less identically. Each wore a stripy shirt, waistcoat with pocket watch and corduroy trousers, usually a mustardy colour. Big boots were the norm, as wellingtons were not as common as they are today. Men and boys carried a stick and would use them if cows or calves got out of control, which was not usual, as cows and calves are a placid lot. Jim Guest was kind to me and would produce his sweet ration from his pocket and give them to me. This band of humans, cows, calves and dogs would process slowly around the area for the whole evening, and the humans would lean over the gate and chat to people as they went by!

On a Saturday we would go to Ross-on-Wye on the midday bus. Everyone was so friendly towards us, greeting us as we got on and enquiring as to my health – so different from when it was thought that I was infectious with tuberculosis. We would visit the grocers, Sadlers, at the bottom of Ross (which is situated on a steep gradient), where you sat on a chair and ordered whatever you could get on your ration book. The place was, I remember, held up with black metal poles which reached to the ceiling. There were scales and bacon slicers, boxes of biscuits and sugar in blue paper bags. The cheese was weighed out and packed in greaseproof paper, with neat folded ends. At Christmas, each family was allowed either a tin of peaches, apricots or pears – not, however, one of each. Overhead ran the money and change dispenser, which went up to the office, where a matriarch woman sat high in her tower office dispensing receipts and change.

We would then walk up the hill to the butchers, Hamblins, which was about halfway up the town. We always went to the same assistant and always had 10/- of beef, lamb or pork. The butcher's name was Fred, and he would reach up high onto the office shelves and give me his sweet ration. By this time I was acquiring quite a stack of sweets, so Mum took charge of them. I am not a glutton for sweets and to this day I can take them or leave them. I suppose it's because I didn't have many in those early post-war years or during my hospitalisation.

I had been discharged from Bristol Hospital in June 1949, but that was not to be my last visit to the hospital. Mum was told that I would need a check-up, blood tests and an X-ray taken every month at first, and then check-ups at less frequent intervals later on, right up until I was twelve years old. Arrangements were made by the hospital.

These visits were to become quite a highlight in my solitary life at Yew Tree Cottage. The appointment for my first check-up was made on my discharge from the hospital. That was to be the first of very many visits. The staff arranged transport for Mum and me for the first few visits. It was either a hospital car or sometimes an ambulance which would pick us up. We would then travel all the way to Bristol, where the driver would wait patiently outside.

Bristol Royal Hospital for Sick Children
OUT-PATIENT DEPT.

Dr. BERYL CORNER

Reg. No.
24331

WEBB. Rosemary

BRING THIS CARD WITH YOU

C40/231/7.63

APPOINTMENTS

23 Jun   1.45
8 Dec   1-45
24 May   1-45
8 Nov   1-45

Outpatient's card
The second card is a later outpatients card with six-monthly
appointments

After these early visits, we were asked if we could go by train and Mum agreed. So from then on an ambulance or car would pick us up from Yew Tree Cottage and take us to Hereford Station, there the driver would buy our train tickets for us and send us on our way on the train. At the other end there would always be another car or ambulance waiting to take us from Temple Meads (Bristol) Station to the hospital. After the tests, X-rays and check-up, the whole process was put into reverse, save that at Hereford we had to walk from the railway station to the ambulance station in Commercial Road (where Morrisons stands today) to order an ambulance to take us home. One night it was snowing badly and the ambulance men tossed a coin to decide who would drive to How Caple and back. Which one won I do not know, but the other driver had a frantic job trying to keep the windscreen clear of snow!

I remember that, on one occasion, we were running late from Bristol Hospital trying to catch train to Hereford when the driver said, 'Hang on, we'll get you there!' He put the bell on to ring, as there were no sirens in those days, and we made it to the train. It was *very* exciting rushing through the centre of Bristol in a blacked-out ambulance with the bell ringing.

As the visits continued, we were asked if we could get up to the hospital at Bristol on our own without a car or ambulance; we could still, however, have our car from Yew Tree Cottage to Hereford station. We agreed to this, and we would usually stop off at Uncle and Auntie's for tea and cake before going on to our appointment. On the return journey, if we stopped off at Uncle and Auntie's, Uncle would fetch me some bananas from his 'plantation' and Auntie would fill our flask for the journey home on the train. On our return to Hereford we would once again go to the ambulance station to order the car or ambulance to take us home.

Isn't it funny what you remember? On one such walk from Bristol Hospital to Temple Meads Station we came upon a policeman guarding a postbox which had overflowed with Christmas cards. It was Christmas Eve, and in those days there was a delivery on Christmas Day.

We sometimes took tea at the Refreshment Room at the station. I absolutely adored Cornish splits and train station tea.

The train we used was the Penzance to Crewe Express (steam) train which passed through Hereford. We didn't have to change trains anywhere. The steam trains drew into Temple Meads in a huge cloud of steam and noise. It was a corridor train with compartments, each seating about eight people. There was always a map on the compartments side and sometimes a couple of pretty pictures of the West Country. There was always a first and third class, why wasn't there a second class? There were toilets on the train but these were never to be used while standing in the station.

I remember vividly the masses of sailors on the train, coming up from Penzance. They were always very kind and played with me, and sometimes, once again, shared their sweets. Their uniforms were always very smart with bell-bottom trousers and horizontal creases all the way up their trouser legs. They were horizontal for the practical purpose of storage, as when the trousers were put away folded up they came out with the creases in them. The sailors also wore a white square of cloth which hung down from the back of the neck like a scarf, over a navy-blue tunic.

The monthly visits to the hospital cheered up my life quite a bit, but I was still very bored and longed to go to school with my friends. Mum was very kind, and as fresh air was still good for me she would drag out the chaise longue into the garden each afternoon so that I could rest and she could read to me, while we both enjoyed the scent from the 'Mrs Sinkins' pinks and the white lilies. It was no mean feat to drag out the chaise longue, as our front door was, to say the least, very awkward. I enjoyed her reading to me, but what I longed to do was read for myself.

During the afternoon ritual of the chaise longue being moved outside, a voice would be heard from the road calling, 'Mrs Webb, are you there?' We would both go down to the road and would find Lady Clive there. Lady Clive was married to General Clive and they both lived at Perrystone Court, about a mile up the road towards Ross. Lady Clive was an invalid and had an invalid carriage, run on batteries. This was a three-wheeled affair and had a wheel at the centre front controlled by a long handle by the lady. From her feet to her waist, she was covered by a waterproof. She would often enquire if I would like to go for a ride. This was gladly accepted and I would sit on the cover to one side of her legs and we would set off and go as far as the Pump Corner and return. Lady Clive went everywhere with that battery-operated chair and she would often go down through the woods towards Foy where there was a wonderful view over the River Wye. There was a seat there which everyone called 'Lady Clive's seat', and in the spring the ground around it was covered in bluebells and primroses.

Eventually the day arrived when I was able to go to school. It was now the autumn of 1949 and I was eight years old, but still unable to read or write. I had to go home to lunch each day in case I was too tired to return for afternoon class. I was so keen, however, that that rarely happened. Dad always came home for lunch wearing the usual workmen's clothes, i.e. stripy shirt with high collar with studs, and he was always losing his studs. He also wore a pair of corduroy trousers and a waistcoat with pockets. He would, during harvest time, and at other times, bring home dead mice in those pockets. He would arrive at lunchtime and our cats, called Kitter and Tinker, would get very excited when he opened the back door and shouted 'Puss, puss', and I would watch in amazement as the cats climbed up my dad and extracted a dead mouse each from his pocket. It was almost a daily ritual. Dad would also, which I now find was illegal, catch baby wild rabbits for me and I would keep them in a hutch in the garden. I adored young things.

When I went back to school, I joined the class with my contemporaries and Mrs Watkins, my teacher, did everything she could to help me.

Bless Mrs Watkins! She could be an ogre at times, but she was very, very patient, and would give the others something to do and then come and sit with me to give me one-to-one tuition. After school, I would stay behind and she would teach me everything she could so that I could 'catch up'. All credit to Mrs Watkins; she tutored me until I knew all the basics and a little bit more. I crammed all I could into my brain and took the eleven-plus exam. Unfortunately I failed the eleven-plus; I suppose I lacked the final polish one needs to get a pass to go to the Grammar School.

After my discharge from hospital and when I was older, during harvest and haymaking times, my mother would, after lunch, put up a basket of sandwiches, cakes and a flask of hot tea for me to take to Dad wherever he was working. This would be after school and could be anywhere on the Chapel Farm and sometimes over a mile away. I would set out with my basket and arrive at the field. At the appropriate time, we would all sit down to tea. Other children brought their dad's tea. When we'd finished, we would play among the sheaves of corn as it was before the combine harvester had been invented. Corn would be placed in stooks ready for collection a couple of weeks later on big trollies. The corn cutting was done with a binder. If it was haymaking time, we would play among the rows of dry, sweet-smelling hay.

I was so happy now, enjoying other children's company and learning the ways of the world, something I'd been denied. I had become very self-reliant, and in a way independent. I would go everywhere with Dad in our little car, accompanying him to work on Saturday and Sundays to feed the stock at the Chapel Farm. Dad loved his animals. There was a secret place at the bottom of the garden at Chapel Farm. A small stream had been 'tamed' to flow through the landscaped garden, about a foot wide, with a pond in the middle. It was 'my place' where I would sit alone on a bench with a book and read for a couple of hours while Dad did his work.

In September 1952 I started at Ross Secondary Modern. The bus picked up at How Caple, then Brockhampton, then Foy and finally arrived at Ross. It was a very long journey in those days, but I did enjoy the ride as well as going to the big modern school. The hospital doctors had told Mum that I was not allowed to do games or swim. I was placed in Class 1B. The placements relied on the Junior School's teacher's report and recommendation, and on Mrs Watkins' direction I had been placed in 1B, and 1A was the class with the brainy children.

About a week after we had been at Ross, we all took another mini test or exam to assess us. We didn't take much notice of this test and forgot all about it, learning to cope with our new lives at this big school and meeting new teachers, doing projects and generally feasting on the new knowledge. Then, horror of horrors, a few days later, Mr Moore (PE and History), who was a giant of a man, read out two names: Carol Stephens and Rosemary Webb. What had we both done? We both shook, as Jasper Moore was not a man to be tangled with.

He said the two of us were to go to Class 1A as we had

been promoted. Class 1A, at that time, was with Miss Betty (English), a quarter of a mile away at the other end of the huge building. Carol and I arrived in Miss Betty's class, where we were told to sit at the back by the window in the two vacant desks. We had met the other two pupils who had been demoted from 1A to 1B en route to our new class.

We knew absolutely no one in this class, only each other. We soon became very firm friends. Carol eventually married Graham, whose career was in banking, and I married a farmer called Gerald. We both have two daughters, and have been devoted friends for the last fifty-six years.

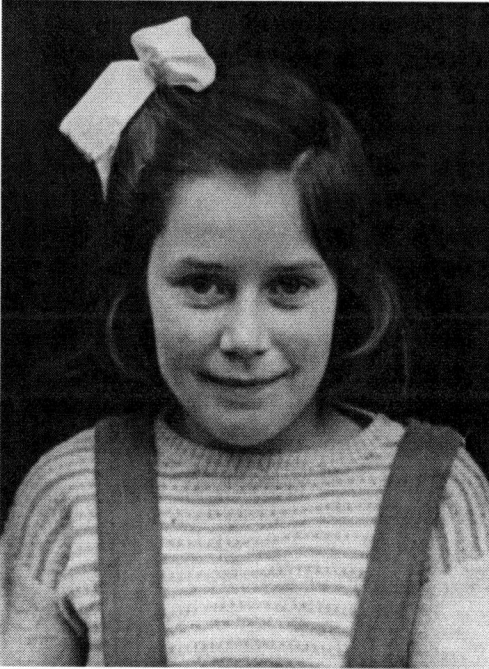

School photo of author

Conclusion

Why have I put down on paper such a traumatic event in my life? Answer: I *needed* to, so that future generations would know what illness, hospital life, expectancy of life with tuberculosis, and recovery rates were in the 1940s.

I was only 5½ years old when I was diagnosed with TB and can only remember snatches of my life then, as most young children can. When do you start to remember events in your very young childhood?

I was taken ill with whooping cough in April 1947, from which I did not recover quickly, and thereafter contracted miliary tuberculosis (TB), supposedly caught from drinking infected milk. Doctors and experts could offer no hope or help from medicine available at the time.

I was nearly six years old when I was admitted to the County Hospital, Hereford, with two months to live, and given penicillin in the hope of curing this dreadful disease, although ideas of a cure were very far from anyone's thoughts, especially the medical professionals.

In September/October 1947 I was moved from the County Hospital for fresh-air treatment at Nieuport Sanatorium, an establishment at Almeley, near Kington, and given up for dead by the medics.

I only spent a few days, or perhaps a week, in Nieuport. Then, in October 1947 I was moved from the Nieuport Sanatorium to Bristol Hospital for Sick Children. The American government had given the English government eighteen beds for treatment using the new 'wonder' drug streptomycin: six in London, six in Birmingham and six in Bristol. This was free of charge, but otherwise it would have cost over £2,000 per head as 1947 was before the dawn of the National Health Service, which came in in 1949. Because a child had died in Bristol, I was given the opportunity to have that precious bed, which was totally free to my mother, father and me.

The Bristol Medical Officer of Health, in his report of 1949, writes:

> It seems a great pity that the results of treatment by streptomycin in experimental animals was so publicised in the press. In actual use on humans, streptomycin has proved rather disappointing. There have been a few dramatic results with TB meningitis, but the number of acute fatal relapses has been very great.

In a report entitled 'The Health of the City of Bristol', of 1949, it is reported that:

> The year 1949 was memorable one if only for the fact that it was the first year of the operation of the National Health Service. Tuberculosis is today the most serious of our infectious diseases – 552 new cases during the year. In other words we are allowing three new cases to appear every two days and the number is going up. There are two deaths every three days.

I was, however, destined not to become one of those statistics in that I lived to tell the tale. Twenty-six months after being taken ill in April 1947, entering the County Hospital in August 1947, being a patient in both the County Hospital and Nieuport Sanatorium, I was discharged fit and well from Bristol Hospital for Sick Children in June 1949.

On reflection now, in the twenty-first century, how cruel and heartless it was to 'snatch' a sick child from its mother and father and place it in hospital with no visitors and no hope of a cure. Such dreadful conditions as

Nieuport House and its horrors should never have been allowed. Twenty-two months of hospitalisation with only sporadic visits by parents and family is unheard of today.

As I say, I have lived to tell the tale, with no lasting side effects, except an intense dislike of hospitals and of being shut in. Apparently streptomycin treatment usually left patients with side effects such as deafness, but thankfully my hearing is OK.

I have tried to capture it all on paper so that future generations can understand what it was like living in the pre-National Health Service era, and then moving into the era of the NHS.

My mother always stated that she and my father were indebted to the American government and the NHS for the cure and treatment which enabled me to lead a more or less normal life.

My dear father, George, who died in 1991, was my soulmate in those post-hospital years and we were very, very close up until his death.

My mother lived to be nearly ninety-four and died early in 2008 and many, many times she relayed to me her fears and worries of those twenty-six months with me being ill at home, in hospital at Hereford, Nieuport, Bristol and Burnham-on-Sea.

However, something happened to prevent any close bonding between the two of us after our forced separation in those formative years. Neither of us could help the circumstances that dragged us apart, but it created a gap between us, never to be closed. I'm afraid that although I loved and respected her dearly, that dreadful time of illness and separation took away that special maternal bond.

I hope my words and recollections are of use to someone in the future, whether for medical research or social history.

Things have moved on so rapidly in medicine since the

1940s and now antibiotics are the norm, but even modern medicines are failing in some quarters.

I will, however, until my death, thank the American government, the wonder drug streptomycin and, of course, the faith of my parents, grandparents and family that enabled me to be cured.

Lightning Source UK Ltd.
Milton Keynes UK
10 February 2010

149848UK00001B/68/P